Epidemiology
and Public Health

NOTICE

Medicine is an ever-changing science. As new research and clinical experience broaden our knowledge, changes in treatment and drug therapy are required. The editors and the publisher of this work have checked with sources believed to be reliable in their efforts to provide information that is complete and generally in accord with the standards accepted at the time of publication. However, in view of the possibility of human error or changes in medical sciences, neither the editors, nor the publisher, nor any other party who has been involved in the preparation or publication of this work warrants that the information contained herein is in every respect accurate or complete. Readers are encouraged to confirm the information contained herein with other sources. For example and in particular, readers are advised to check the product information sheet included in the package of each drug they plan to administer to be certain that the information contained in this book is accurate and that changes have not been made in the recommended dose or in the contraindications for administration. This recommendation is of particular importance in connection with new or infrequently used drugs.

Epidemiology and Public Health

PreTest® Self-Assessment and Review

Fifth Edition

Edited by

Thomas B. Newman, M.D., M.P.H.

Assistant Professor of Pediatrics and Epidemiology
University of California at San Francisco
San Francisco, California

Warren S. Browner, M.D., M.P.H.

Assistant Professor of Medicine and Epidemiology
University of California at San Francisco
San Francisco, California

McGraw-Hill Information Services Company
Health Professions Division
PreTest Series

New York St. Louis San Francisco Colorado Springs Auckland Bogotá Hamburg
Lisbon London Madrid Mexico Milan Montreal New Delhi Panama Paris
San Juan São Paulo Singapore Sydney Tokyo Toronto

Library of Congress Cataloging-in-Publication Data

Epidemiology and public health : PreTest self-assessment and review.—
  5th ed. / edited by Thomas B. Newman, Warren S. Browner.
    p.   cm.
  Bibliography: p.
  ISBN 0-07-051972-2 : $14.95
    1. Public health—Examinations, questions, etc.   2. Epidemiology—
Examinations, questions, etc.   I. Newman, Thomas B.   II. Browner,
Warren S.
    [DNLM: 1. Epidemiology—examination questions.   2. Public
Health—examination questions.   WA 18 E643]
RA430.E65   1989
362.1'076—dc19
DNLM/DLC
for Library of Congress   89-2732
                                                                   CIP

This book was set in Times Roman by Waldman Graphics, Inc.; the editors
were J. Dereck Jeffers and Bruce MacGregor; the production supervisor was
Clara B. Stanley.
R. R. Donnelley & Sons was printer and binder.

1 2 3 4 5 6 7 8 9 0   DOCDOC   8 9 4 3 2 1 0 9

ISBN 0-07-051972-2

Contents

Introduction   vii

Principles and Methods of Epidemiology
  Questions   1
  Answers, Explanations, and References   23

Communicable Diseases
  Questions   43
  Answers, Explanations, and References   59

Chronic Diseases
  Questions   79
  Answers, Explanations, and References   92

Occupational and Environmental Health
  Questions   105
  Answers, Explanations, and References   118

Mental Health
  Questions   134
  Answers, Explanations, and References   144

Community Medicine
  Questions   155
  Answers, Explanations, and References   164

Health Care Delivery Systems
  Questions   174
  Answers, Explanations, and References   180

Bibliography   185

Introduction

Epidemiology and Public Health, PreTest Self-Assessment and Review, 5th Ed., has been designed to provide medical students, as well as physicians, with a comprehensive and convenient instrument for self-assessment and review within the field of epidemiology and public health. The 500 questions provided have been designed to parallel the format and degree of difficulty of the questions contained in Part II of the National Board of Medical Examiners examinations, the Federation Licensing Examination (FLEX), and the Foreign Medical Graduate Examination in the Medical Sciences (FMGEMS).

Each question in the book is accompanied by an answer, a paragraph explanation, and a specific page reference to either a current journal article, a textbook, or both. A bibliography that lists all the sources used in the book follows the last chapter.

Perhaps the most effective way to use this book is to allow yourself one minute to answer each question in a given chapter; as you proceed, indicate your answer beside each question. By following this suggestion, you will be approximating the time limits imposed by the board examinations previously mentioned.

When you have finished answering the questions in a chapter, you should then spend as much time as you need verifying your answers and carefully reading the explanations. Although you should pay special attention to the explanations for the questions you answered incorrectly, you should read every explanation. The authors of this book have designed the explanations to reinforce and supplement the information tested by the questions. If, after reading the explanations for a given chapter, you feel you need still more information about the material covered, you should consult and study the references indicated.

Epidemiology
and Public Health

Principles and Methods of Epidemiology

DIRECTIONS: Each question below contains five suggested responses. Select the **one best** response to each question.

1. Epidemiology can be defined as the study of

(A) the etiology of disease in humans
(B) the frequency of causes of death in humans
(C) the determinants of frequency of disease in humans
(D) the distribution and determinants of frequency of disease in humans
(E) the patterns of organization and financing of health care

2. A sample of 1,000 people includes 120 who are hearing-impaired and 50 who are diabetic. If the number who are both diabetic and hearing impaired is 6, then

(A) diabetes and hearing impairment appear to be independent characteristics
(B) diabetics appear to be protected from hearing impairment
(C) diabetics appear to be at greater risk of hearing impairment
(D) there is an interaction between diabetes and hearing impairment
(E) there is not sufficient information to state any of the above

3. A measure of the amount of variation of a set of values about the mean is the

(A) regression coefficient
(B) standard error of the mean
(C) standard deviation
(D) range
(E) correlation coefficient

4. The association between low birth weight and maternal smoking during pregnancy can be studied by obtaining smoking histories from women at the time of their prenatal visit and then subsequently correlating birth weight with smoking histories. What type of study is this?

(A) Clinical trial
(B) Cross-sectional
(C) Cohort (prospective)
(D) Case-control (retrospective)
(E) None of the above

5. An investigator wishes to perform a randomized clinical trial to evaluate a new beta-blocker as a treatment for hypertension. To be eligible for the study, subjects must have a resting diastolic blood pressure of at least 90 mmHg. One hundred patients seen at the screening clinic with this level of hypertension are recruited for the study and make appointments with the study nurse. When the nurse obtains their blood pressure 2 weeks later, only 65 of them have diastolic blood pressures of 90 mmHg or more. The most likely explanation for this is

(A) spontaneous resolution
(B) regression toward the mean
(C) baseline drift
(D) measurement error
(E) Hawthorne effect

6. A study is undertaken to determine whether use of Newman and Browner's *PreTest Self-Assessment and Review* reduces sexual dysfunction related to anxiety before board examinations. One group of students studying for their board examinations was given the book to read; the other was not. The results are as follows:

Outcome	Got Book	Did Not Get Book
Sexual dysfunction	3	34
No sexual dysfunction	61	32

All the following statements are true EXCEPT

(A) these data could be analyzed using the chi-square test
(B) about half of the control group experienced sexual dysfunction
(C) unless one knows on what basis group assignment was made (i.e., randomized or not), the results are difficult to interpret
(D) the difference is probably due to chance
(E) a t test is inappropriate to analyze the data because the variables are categorical rather than continuous

7. Reye syndrome is an acute encephalopathy of childhood, accompanied by fatty infiltration of the liver. It has been linked to use of aspirin during infections with chickenpox or influenza. Children commonly progress through a sequence of stages that are used to grade severity and prognosis. If 30 percent of children progress only to stage I, 40 percent only to stage II, 20 percent only to stage III, and 10 percent to stage IV, what is the probability that a child will progress to stage IV, once that child has already reached stage II?

(A) 10 percent
(B) 14 percent
(C) 30 percent
(D) 33 percent
(E) None of the above

8. If the chance of acquiring serologic evidence of human immunodeficiency virus (HIV) from an infected sexual partner is a constant 30 percent per year, what is the approximate chance of becoming infected within 3 years?

(A) 10 percent
(B) 30 percent
(C) 66 percent
(D) 90 percent
(E) None of the above

9. Which of the following measures is used frequently as a denominator to calculate the incidence rate of a disease?

(A) Number of cases observed
(B) Number of new cases observed
(C) Number of asymptomatic cases
(D) Person-years of observation
(E) Persons lost to follow-up

10. In 1971, the crude birth rate in the United States was approximately 17 per 1,000 population; the death rate was 10 per 1,000; and the net in-migration rate was 2 per 1,000. What was the net growth rate per 1,000?

(A) 5
(B) 7
(C) 9
(D) 15
(E) 25

11. In nine families surveyed, the numbers of children per family were 4, 6, 2, 2, 4, 3, 2, 1, 7. The mean, median, and mode numbers of children per family are

(A) 3.4, 2, 3
(B) 3, 3.4, 2
(C) 3, 3, 2
(D) 2, 3.5, 3
(E) none of the above

Questions 12–14

The results of a study of the incidence of pulmonary tuberculosis in a village in India are given in the table below. All persons in the village are examined during two surveys made 2 years apart, and the number of new cases was used to determine the incidence rate.

Category of Household at First Survey	Number of Persons	Number of New Cases
With culture-positive case	500	10
Without culture-positive case	10,000	10

12. What is the incidence of new cases per 1,000 person-years in households that had a culture-positive case during the first survey?

(A) 0.02
(B) 0.01
(C) 1.0
(D) 10
(E) 20

13. What is the incidence of new cases per 1,000 person-years in households that did not have a culture-positive case during the first survey?

(A) 0.001
(B) 0.1
(C) 0.5
(D) 1.0
(E) 5.0

14. What is the relative risk of acquiring tuberculosis in households with a culture-positive case compared with households without tuberculosis?

(A) 0.05
(B) 0.5
(C) 2.0
(D) 10
(E) 20

15. During the investigation of an outbreak of food poisoning at a summer camp, food histories were obtained from all campers as indicated in the table below. Which of the food items was probably responsible for the outbreak?

| | Food | Proportion Ill (Percent) | |
		Campers Who Ate Specified Food	Campers Who Did Not Eat Specified Food
(A)	Hamburger	61	48
(B)	Potatoes	70	35
(C)	Ice cream	40	50
(D)	Chicken	73	10
(E)	Lemonade	20	45

16. Which of the following statements concerning statistical inference is correct?

(A) If the p value = 0.05, then there is a 95 percent probability that the results did not occur by chance

(B) The null hypothesis generally states that there is a difference between the groups

(C) If the p value is sufficiently high, the null hypothesis is not rejected

(D) Knowledge of the sampling method is not important in determining statistical significance

(E) None of the above

17. In the study of the cause of a disease, the essential difference between an *experimental* study and an *observational* study is that in the experimental investigation

(A) the study is prospective

(B) the study is retrospective

(C) the study and control groups are of equal size

(D) the study and control groups are selected on the basis of history of exposure to the suspected causal factor

(E) the investigators determine who is and who is not exposed to the suspected causal factor

Questions 18–19

To determine whether prenatal exposure to tobacco smoke is a cause of undescended testes in newborns, the mothers of 100 newborns with undescended testes and 100 newborns whose testes had descended were questioned about smoking habits during pregnancy. The study revealed an odds ratio of 2.6 associated with exposure to smoke, with 95 percent confidence intervals from 1.1 to 5.3.

18. Which of the following statements is true?

(A) The odds ratio could be falsely elevated by the inclusion of infants whose testes were descended (but retractile) in the case group (misclassification bias)

(B) The odds ratio could be falsely elevated by recall bias if parents of affected infants were more likely to remember or report their exposures

(C) Because the cases are newborns, but the exposure data came from their mothers, this is not a true case-control study

(D) Since the study was not blinded, it is impossible to rule out a placebo effect

(E) None of the above

19. Which of the following statements is true?

(A) The results provide no evidence that maternal cigarette smoking is associated with undescended testes in the offspring

(B) If the study results are accurate, they suggest that a baby boy whose mother smoked is about 2.6 times as likely to be born with testes undescended as a baby boy whose mother did not smoke

(C) The fact that the confidence interval excludes 1 indicates that $p > .05$

(D) The 90 percent confidence interval for these results would probably include 1.0

(E) None of the above

20. In order to determine the relationship between serum levels of sodium and antidiuretic hormone (ADH) in patients who have meningitis, the most appropriate study design would be

(A) repeated measurement of sodium and ADH in a patient with meningitis

(B) measurement of both sodium and ADH in a set of patients with meningitis

(C) measurements of sodium in one set of patients and of ADH in a different set of patients

(D) measurements of ADH in a set of patients with meningitis and a set of controls with other illnesses

(E) none of the above

21. The probability of being born with condition A is 0.10 and the probability of being born with condition B is 0.50. If conditions A and B are independent, what is the probability of being born with either condition A or condition B (or both)?

(A) 0.05
(B) 0.40
(C) 0.50
(D) 0.55
(E) 0.60

22. All the following are important steps in decision analysis EXCEPT

(A) construction of a decision tree
(B) estimation of probabilities at chance nodes
(C) assignment of utilities
(D) estimation of sample size
(E) determination of how changes in probability estimates affect the decision

23. All the following statements regarding the normal (Gaussian) distribution are true EXCEPT

(A) the mean = median = mode
(B) approximately 50 percent of observations are greater than the mode
(C) approximately 68 percent of observations fall within 1 standard deviation of the mean
(D) the number of observations between 0 and 1 standard deviation from the mean is the same as the number between 1 and 2 standard deviations from the mean
(E) the shape of the curve does not depend on the value of the mean

Questions 24–26

Lou Stewells, a pioneer in the study of diarrheal disease, has developed a new diagnostic test for cholera. When his agent is added to the stool, the organisms develop a characteristic ring around them. (He calls it the "Ring-Around-the-Cholera" [RAC] test.) He performs the test on 100 patients known to have cholera and 100 patients known not to have cholera with the following results:

	Cholera	No Cholera
RAC test +	91	12
RAC test −	9	88
Totals	100	100

24. All the following statements about the RAC test are correct EXCEPT

(A) the sensitivity of the test was about 91 percent
(B) the specificity of the test was about 12 percent
(C) the false negative rate was about 9 percent
(D) the predictive value of a positive result cannot be determined from the above
(E) the predictive value of a negative result cannot be determined from the above

25. Dr. Stewells next performs the test on 1,000 patients admitted to the hospital with profuse diarrhea. The results are as follows:

	Cholera	No Cholera
RAC test +	312	79
RAC test −	31	578
Totals	343	657

Which of the following statements is correct?

(A) The predictive value of a positive result is 312/343
(B) The predictive value of a positive result is 79/312
(C) The predictive value of a negative result is 578/(578 + 31)
(D) The incidence rate of cholera in this population is 343/1,000
(E) None of the above

26. After many years and dozens of publications, the RAC test achieves widespread acceptance, and Dr. Stewells' position in the Diarrhea Hall of Fame seems assured. However, with improvements in hygiene, the prevalence of cholera gradually falls from the high of about 35 percent of hospitalized diarrhea patients to only 5 percent. Which of the following statements about the effect of this fall in prevalence is true?

(A) The change in prevalence will reduce the predictive value of a negative result
(B) The predictive value of a positive result will decline
(C) The specificity of the test is likely to decline
(D) The specificity of the test will increase at the expense of its sensitivity
(E) None of the above

27. Randomization is a procedure used for assignment or allocation of subjects to treatment and control groups in experimental studies. Randomization ensures

(A) that assignment occurs by chance
(B) that treatment and control groups are alike in all respects except treatment
(C) that bias in observations is eliminated
(D) that placebo effects are eliminated
(E) none of the above

28. In comparing the difference between two means, the value of p is found to be 0.60. The correct interpretation of this result is

(A) the null hypothesis is rejected
(B) the difference is statistically significant
(C) the difference occurred by chance
(D) the difference is compatible with the null hypothesis
(E) sampling variation is an unlikely explanation of the difference

29. In a study of the cause of lung cancer, patients who had the disease were matched with controls by age, sex, place of residence, and social class. The frequency of cigarette smoking was then compared in the two groups. What type of study was this?

(A) Cohort (prospective)
(B) Case-control (retrospective)
(C) Clinical trial
(D) Historical cohort
(E) None of the above

30. In country A there are 35 new cases of breast cancer per 100,000 adult women per year; in country B the number is 90 per 100,000. Which of the following is the most likely explanation?

(A) Women in country A have a much higher rate of nursing their infants
(B) Women in country A are less likely to smoke cigarettes
(C) Women in country A receive more frequent preventive care, such as mammography
(D) Treatment is much more successful in country A
(E) Women in country A are younger

Questions 31–33

Smoking and alcohol use are both risk factors for esophageal cancer. The hypothetical table below shows how the incidence of esophageal cancer varies with either smoking or alcohol use (but not both):

	Incidence (cases/10,000 person-yr)	
	Nonsmoker	Smoker
Nondrinker	10	50
Drinker	30	X

31. All the following statements are true EXCEPT

(A) in nonsmokers, the excess risk of esophageal cancer from drinking is 20 cases per 10,000 person-years
(B) in nondrinkers, the relative risk of esophageal cancer from smoking is 5.0
(C) the overall relative risk for smoking cannot be determined without knowledge of X and the proportion of the population that drinks
(D) the table shows that smoking causes more cases of esophageal cancer in this population than does drinking
(E) in nondrinkers, the excess risk of esophageal cancer from smoking is 40 cases per 10,000 person-years

32. If smoking and alcohol act independently to cause esophageal cancer under an *additive* model, what would be the expected value of X?

(A) 60
(B) 70
(C) 80
(D) 150
(E) None of the above

33. If smoking and alcohol act independently according to a *multiplicative* model, what would be the expected value of X?

(A) 70
(B) 80
(C) 120
(D) 1500
(E) None of the above

DIRECTIONS: Each question below contains four suggested responses of which **one or more** is correct. Select

A	if	**1, 2, and 3**	are correct
B	if	**1 and 3**	are correct
C	if	**2 and 4**	are correct
D	if	**4**	is correct
E	if	**1, 2, 3, and 4**	are correct

34. When direct, controlled experiments cannot be performed, the determination of whether or not an association between events is causal must rest on observational data. Which of the following types of evidence can be used in judging whether or not a cause-and-effect relationship between events exists?

(1) Strength of the association
(2) Consistency of the association in different studies
(3) Proper time sequence in which putative cause precedes effect
(4) Consistency of a causal association with existing knowledge

---

SUMMARY OF DIRECTIONS

A	B	C	D	E
1,2,3	1,3	2,4	4	All are
only	only	only	only	correct

---

35. In the table below, data are presented on the number of children suffering from acute leukemia who were admitted to a hospital between 1970 and 1984. Correct conclusions about the data include which of the following?

Age (years)	Number of Children Admitted in Interval		
	1970–74	1975–79	1980–84
0–4	12	23	31
5–9	8	17	36
10–14	10	7	4
Total	30	47	71

(1) The incidence of leukemia decreased in children 10 to 14 years old

(2) The prevalence of leukemia increased in children between 1970 and 1984

(3) The incidence of leukemia increased in children 5 to 9 years old

(4) The number of children 9 years old and under admitted to the study hospital because of acute leukemia increased between 1970 and 1984

36. The *attributable risk* of a disease estimates the maximum proportion of the disease in the population attributable to a particular risk factor. For example, in the U.S., the attributable risk of lung cancer from active smoking is about 85 percent; this means that active smoking may explain up to 85 percent of the cases of lung cancer that occur in the U.S. For a particular disease and risk factor, the attributable risk depends on

(1) the size of the population of interest
(2) the prevalence of the risk factor in the population
(3) the duration of the disease
(4) the relative risk (risk ratio) of the disease associated with the risk factor

37. Correct statements concerning statistical inference include which of the following?

(1) If the p value is very low, the difference between the groups must be very large
(2) The standard error of the mean is used to estimate how closely the mean of a sample approximates the true population mean
(3) If the sample size is large enough, it is easy to achieve statistical significance at the 0.05 level, even when there is no difference between the groups
(4) All else being equal, use of one-tailed rather than two-tailed tests of statistical significance will more often lead to rejecting the null hypothesis when it is true

38. A randomized, double-blinded trial finds that oral corticosteroids are superior to placebo in hastening the resolution of otitis media with effusion. Possible reasons why this study might have given a falsely positive result include

(1) it may be difficult accurately to determine which effusions have resolved, leading to errors in determining the outcome of the study
(2) lax inclusion criteria may have led to inclusion of some subjects in the study who did not really have otitis media with effusion
(3) the sample size may have been too small
(4) the apparent effect might be a result of chance

39. An investigator is designing a randomized clinical trial to see whether vitamin E will prevent cancer in smokers. Which of the following would be important considerations in planning the sample size for the study?

(1) The expected incidence of cancer in the placebo group
(2) The frequency with which subjects are likely to be lost to follow-up or die from noncancer causes over the duration of the study
(3) The magnitude of the preventive effect that the investigator wishes to be able to detect
(4) The values for alpha and beta, the type 1 and type 2 error rates

40. According to the report form (U.S. Standard Report of Fetal Death) recommended by the National Center for Health Statistics, facts required in completing a report of a fetal death include which of the following?

(1) Weight of fetus
(2) The month in the pregnancy when prenatal care began
(3) Complications of labor
(4) Whether an autopsy was performed

41. Investigators determine that a statistically significant difference exists between the incidences of a disease in two groups of subjects. This significant difference may be the result of

(1) causal association
(2) chance association
(3) indirect association
(4) artifactual association

42. In a study of level of blood lead as a predictor of IQ in children, a simple linear regression analysis is performed. The regression coefficient for lead is -0.1 IQ points per μg Pb/dl blood. The coefficient is highly statistically significant ($p < .001$). Correct conclusions include which of the following?

(1) The relationship between blood lead and IQ is linear
(2) Lead causes a decrease in the IQ in children of about 0.1 point for each μg/dl of blood lead
(3) The study provides convincing evidence that lead and IQ are independently associated
(4) All else being equal, the expected difference in IQ between two children whose lead levels differ by 50 μg/dl is about 5 points

43. Correct statements about infant mortality include which of the following?

(1) The numerator is the number of deaths of infants in the first month of life
(2) The rate is expressed per 1,000 live births.
(3) In the U.S., the single most important cause of infant mortality is sudden infant death syndrome (SIDS)
(4) In the U.S., infant mortality is about twice as high in blacks as in whites

44. When selecting the control group to be used in a case-control study, one must

(1) be assured that information on study factors can be obtained from controls in a manner similar to that by which it was obtained from cases

(2) consider whether or not to match the controls in such a way as to make them similar to the cases with respect to confounding variables

(3) understand it is desirable that the controls be derived from a population generally similar to that which gave rise to the case

(4) take into account a variety of practical and economic considerations

45. True statements concerning cohort studies include which of the following?

(1) Cohort studies are longitudinal in design

(2) Subjects are selected on the basis of characteristics present before the onset of the condition being studied

(3) Subjects are observed over time to determine the frequency of occurrence of the condition under study

(4) They are primarily descriptive, rather than analytic

46. For many diagnostic or screening tests, there is a tradeoff between sensitivity and specificity. True statements include which of the following?

(1) Sensitivity would be extremely important when testing for amyotrophic lateral sclerosis (ALS) because there is no good treatment for it

(2) Because hypothyroidism in infancy is devastating if missed, a screening test for it should be highly specific

(3) Specificity is more important than sensitivity for screening tests

(4) In evaluating the potential usefulness of a screening test, the effectiveness of treatment for the disease screened for is of great importance

47. Which of the following assumptions must be satisfied in order to apply the student t test to analyze the statistical significance of the difference between two sample means?

(1) The samples must be independent

(2) The standard deviations of the populations being sampled must be approximately equal

(3) The samples must be normally distributed

(4) The samples must be equal in size

DIRECTIONS: Each group of questions below consists of lettered headings followed by a set of numbered items. For each numbered item select the **one** lettered heading with which it is **most** closely associated. Each lettered heading may be used **once, more than once, or not at all.**

Questions 48–51

For each of the studies below, choose the most appropriate statistical test to analyze the data.

(A) Chi-square analysis
(B) Student t test
(C) Analysis of variance
(D) Paired t test
(E) Linear regression

48. Comparison of systolic blood pressures in independent samples of pregnant and nonpregnant women

49. Comparison of the prevalence of hepatitis B surface antigen (HBsAg) in medical and dental students

50. Comparison of the level of blood glucose in male and female rats following administration of three different drugs

51. Comparison of serum cholesterol before and after ingestion of hamburgers in a sample of fast-food patrons

Questions 52–55

In each statement below, data are presented based on a cohort study of coronary heart disease. Choose the parameter that best describes each of these statements.

(A) Point prevalence
(B) Incidence rate
(C) Standardized morbidity ratio
(D) Relative risk
(E) None of the above

52. At the initial examination, 17 persons per 1,000 had evidence of coronary heart disease (CHD)

53. Among heavy smokers, the observed frequency of angina pectoris was 1.6 times as great as the expected frequency during the first 12 years of the study

54. During the first 8 years of the study, 45 persons developed coronary heart disease per 1,000 persons who entered the study free of disease

55. The risk of coronary heart disease was 23 percent higher in relatives of patients with CHD than in the general population

Questions 56–59

Choose the rate that best describes each statement below.

(A) Secondary attack rate
(B) Case-fatality rate
(C) Morbidity rate
(D) Age-adjusted mortality
(E) Crude mortality

56. Death occurs in 10 percent of cases of meningococcal meningitis

57. Approximately 9 people die each year in the United States for every 1,000 estimated to be alive

58. Eighty percent of susceptible household contacts of a child with chickenpox develop this disease

59. Children between the ages of 1 and 5 have an average of eight colds per year

Questions 60–63

For each of the descriptions of statistical procedures below, choose the statistical error.

(A) Observations are not independent

(B) Variable is not normally distributed

(C) Unequal group sizes or unequal variances

(D) Not enough degrees of freedom

(E) None of the above

60. The frequencies of infection of the urinary tract are compared in 24 children treated with intermittent catheterization and 9 children treated with urinary diversion. In the catheterization group 85/231 urine cultures were positive, compared with 34/55 in the diversion group. The difference between these two proportions was statistically significant ($X^2 = 11.4$, degrees of freedom = 1, p < .001)

61. The mean lengths of hospital stay were compared in 34 patients treated surgically and 34 patients treated medically for acute peritonsillar abscess. The mean lengths of stay in the two groups were 4.3 ± 3.1 and 2.7 ± 3.1 (mean $\pm$ standard deviation), respectively. The t test was significant ($t = 2.13$, p = .05)

62. The parity of 100 women with breast cancer was compared with that of 200 controls. Among the cases, 40 percent were nulliparous, 30 percent had one child, and 30 percent had more than one child; among the controls the numbers were 20, 30, and 50 percent, respectively. The mean ($\pm$ SD) parity in the cases was 1.6 ± 2.1; in the controls it was 2.2 ± 2.3. The difference was statistically significant using the t test ($t = -2.2$; p = 0.04)

63. An investigator wishes to examine the efficacy of varicella vaccine. For convenience, he randomizes four classes of third graders for the study: two classes receive the vaccine, and two do not. Over the next year, only 2/57 children in the vaccine group, but 25/60 children in the control group get chickenpox ($X^2 = 23$, degrees of freedom = 1, p < .001). The investigator concludes that the vaccine is highly effective

Questions 64–67

For each of the studies described below, select the critical statement that best explains why the conclusion is misleading or false.

(A) Lack of a control group
(B) Lack of proper follow-up
(C) Lack of adjustment for age
(D) Lack of denominators
(E) Lack of adjustment for race

64. Of 250 consecutive, unselected women in whom acute cholecystitis was diagnosed, 75 of these women were under age 50 and 175 were over age 50. The investigator concluded that acute cholecystitis is more common in postmenopausal women

65. In a review of 3,000 patients in whom adult-onset diabetes was diagnosed, 2,000 of these patients were obese at the time of diagnosis. The investigator concluded that there was an association between diabetes and obesity

66. Acute anxiety neurosis was diagnosed among 250 patients and follow-up data were available on 80 percent of these patients 10 years later. The mortality experience of this cohort was no different than that of the general population. The authors concluded that the diagnosis of acute anxiety neurosis was not associated with a decrease in longevity

67. Among 143 patients dying of bacterial endocarditis on whom autopsies were performed, 2 percent of patients were less than 10 years of age. The authors concluded that bacterial endocarditis is rare in childhood

Questions 68–71

Choose the term that best fits the description.

(A) Matching
(B) Stratification
(C) Age adjustment
(D) Multivariate statistical analysis
(E) Survival analysis

68. In a cohort study of hypertensive men, the proportions of subjects with high and low renin levels who survived for 5 years are compared separately among those aged 40 to 49, those aged 50 to 59, and those aged 60 to 69 at entry

69. A sampling strategy is used to achieve comparability of the groups being studied

70. A technique takes into account variable length of follow-up

71. Six different risk ratios are calculated: one for each sex at each of three social class levels

Questions 72–75

The following two-by-two table represents the findings of a 5-year cohort study in which the incidence of suicide in veterans who served in Vietnam was compared with that of veterans who served elsewhere. Match the name of the parameter below with the appropriate formula.

	Suicide	No Suicide
Served in Vietnam	a	b
Served elsewhere	c	d

(A) ad/bc
(B) (a + b)/(a + b + c + d)
(C) (a + c)/(a + b + c + d)
(D) [a/(a + b)]/[c/(c + d)]
(E) a/(a + b) − c/(c + d)

72. The odds ratio

73. The relative risk

74. The excess risk of suicide in Vietnam veterans

75. The overall incidence (per 5 years) of suicide in the study

Questions 76–79

Match each description of a sampling procedure with the correct term.

(A) Systematic sampling
(B) Paired sampling
(C) Simple random sampling
(D) Stratified sampling
(E) Cluster sampling

76. Each individual of the total group has an equal chance of being selected

77. Households are selected at random, and every person in each household is included in the sample

78. Individuals are initially assembled according to some order in a group and then individuals are selected according to some constant determinant; e.g., every fourth subject is selected

79. Individuals are divided into subgroups on the basis of specified characteristics and then random samples are selected from each subgroup

Questions 80–82

For each disease or condition, select the best available source of information.

(A) Death certificates
(B) Household surveys
(C) Cancer registry
(D) State health department
(E) Life insurance companies

80. Incidence of meningococcal meningitis in Connecticut

81. Prevalence of arthritis

82. Survival rate of patients with cancer of the pancreas

Questions 83–86

Select the letter corresponding to the figure that best fits each description.

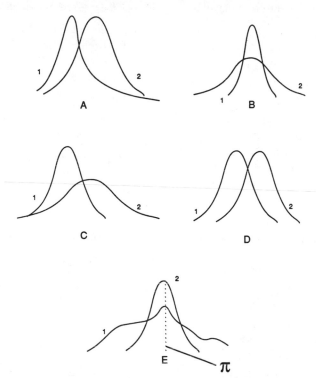

83. Distributions 1 and 2 have the same median and mean, but 2 has the greater variance

84. Distributions 1 and 2 have the same variance, but different means

85. Compared with curve 2, curve 1 is skewed to the right

86. This figure represents a tasty dessert

Questions 87–90

For each result or conclusion described below, select the choice that might best explain it.

(A) Ecologic fallacy
(B) Type 1 error
(C) Type 2 error
(D) Selection bias
(E) Misclassification bias

87. A randomized blinded trial of aspirin to prevent myocardial infarction fails to find a difference between aspirin and placebo groups after 5 years (N = 500 per group; p = .11)

88. A study of patterns of contraceptive use finds that counties with the highest per-capita use of condoms also have the highest pregnancy rates (N = 100,000; p < .001) and concludes that condoms are ineffective as contraceptives

89. An investigator analyzes data from the National Health Interview Survey and finds that there is a positive association between consumption of turkey and degenerative joint disease (N = 5000; p < .05).

90. In a case-control study of lung cancer, cases' spouses are chosen as controls. The odds ratio for smoking is 3.0, which does not quite reach statistical significance (N = 30 per group; p = .07).

Questions 91–95

For each variable described below, choose the type of measurement scale.

(A) Dichotomous scale
(B) Nominal scale
(C) Ordinal scale
(D) Interval scale
(E) Ratio scale

91. Survival of a particular patient for at least 5 years

92. Frequency of somnolence during biochemistry lectures: never, sometimes, usually, or always

93. Birth weight

94. Type of medical specialty

95. Year of birth

Principles and Methods of Epidemiology

Answers

1. The answer is D. *(Mausner, ed 2. p 1.)* The word *epidemiology* comes from the Greek words *epi* (upon) and *demos* (people). In fact, there is a separate word for the study of determinants of disease in animals—*epizootiology*. Epidemiology is the study of both the distribution of diseases in human populations and the determinants of the observed distribution. It began as the study of infectious diseases but has expanded to include the study of chronic diseases, organization of health care, delivery of health care, and occupational and environmental health.

2. The answer is A. *(Ingelfinger, ed 2. pp 11–12.)* Two characteristics are independent of each other (i.e., unrelated) if and only if the probability of both occurring in the same person is equal to the product of their probabilities. In this example, we estimate the probability of hearing impairment in this population as $120/1,000 = 0.12$, and the probability of diabetes as $50/1,000 = 0.05$. The product of these probabilities is $(.12)(.05) = 0.006$. Thus, with a sample of size 1,000, if hearing impairment and diabetes were independent, we would expect about 6 persons to be both hearing impaired and diabetic—exactly what was found.

3. The answer is C. *(Colton, pp 31, 189–195.)* The *standard deviation (SD)* is a measure of the variability or scatter of a set of observations about the mean. A large SD means that the observations are widely scattered about the mean, whereas a small SD indicates that they are clustered closely about the mean. The *standard error of the mean (SEM)* is a measure of the variability of a sample mean. Thus, whereas the SD reflects scatter of observations about the (sample or population) mean, the SEM reflects scatter of sample means around the true population mean. The larger the sample, the closer its mean is likely to be to the population mean. Thus, as the sample size increases, the standard error of the mean decreases. Mathematically, the SEM is equal to the sample standard deviation divided by the square-root of the sample size $(SD/\sqrt{n})$. The *range* describes the variability only in terms of the smallest and largest values without indicating the distribution of the values about the mean. The *regression* and *correlation coefficients* are measures of the degree of relationship between two variables.

4.   The answer is C. *(Mausner, ed 2. pp 156–158.)* This study is a *cohort* (prospective) study because the subjects (pregnant women) were categorized on the basis of exposure or lack of exposure to a risk factor (smoking during pregnancy), and then were followed to determine if the outcome (low-birth-weight babies) resulted. The term *cohort* refers to the group of subjects who are followed forward in time to see which ones develop the outcome. *Clinical trials* are prospective studies in which an *intervention* is applied—no intervention was mentioned in the question. In a *case-control* (retrospective) study of the relationship between low birth weight and maternal smoking, infants would be selected on the basis of low birth weight (cases) and normal birth weight (controls) and then the frequency of maternal smoking would be compared in the two groups. In *cross-sectional* studies exposure and outcome are measured at the same point in time.

5.   The answer is B. *(Ingelfinger, ed 2. pp 189–191.)* Although hypertension can resolve spontaneously, this is an unlikely explanation for resolution over a 2-week period in 35 percent of the subjects. A much more likely explanation is *regression toward the mean*. Because of random fluctuations, any one measurement of blood pressure may be far from a person's normal blood pressure. By referring patients for the study based on a single measurement, those in whom the measurement was falsely high are much more likely to be referred than those in whom the measurement was too low. Thus in any group selected based on a characteristic with substantial day-to-day variation, many will have values closer to the population mean when the measurement is repeated. Neither baseline drift (which occurs with measurements on certain machines requiring frequent calibration) nor measurement error is as likely an explanation. The Hawthorne effect refers to a tendency among study subjects to change simply because they are being studied. It is much more likely to affect studies of behavior or attitudes than a study of blood pressure.

6.   The answer is D. *(Colton, pp 129, 174.)* The data presented are for a dichotomous predictor variable (book/no book) and a dichotomous outcome variable (dysfunction/no dysfunction), so a chi-square test (but not a t test) is appropriate for analysis. Since there is apparently such a big difference between the groups, chance is not a likely explanation for the findings. It is essential to know how the groups were assigned if the study is to be properly interpreted. In fact, in this case, we chose the control group from subjects at a clinic for sexual dysfunction.

7.   The answer is B. *(Colton, pp 71–73.)* The overall probability of reaching stage IV is 10 percent; i.e., of 100 patients, about 10 would be expected to reach stage IV. However, if it is given that the patient has reached stage II, that patient has missed his or her chance to stop at stage I, so the probability of reaching stage IV is a little greater. In fact, since 30 of 100 patients get no farther than stage I, only 70 make it to stage II or more. Of these, 10 will make it to stage IV. The probability of reaching stage IV given that one has reached stage II is thus about 10/70 (14 percent).

8.   The answer is C. *(Ingelfinger, ed 2. pp 37–46.)* The chance of remaining uninfected for 1 year is 0.7; for 3 years it is (0.7) (0.7) (0.7) = 0.343. Everyone who does not remain uninfected must become infected; thus the chance of becoming infected is 1 − 0.343 = 0.657, or about 66 percent.

9.   The answer is D. *(Mausner, ed 2. pp 46–48.)* Person-years of observation are frequently used in the denominator of incidence rates and provide a method of dealing with variable follow-up periods. Person-years of observation simultaneously take into account the number of persons under observation and the duration of observation of each person. For example, if 8 new cases of diabetes occurred among 1,000 people followed for 2 years, the incidence would be 8 cases per 2,000 person-years, or 4 per 1,000 person-years of follow-up. The distinction between *rates* and *proportions* is not well maintained in standard epidemiologic terminology. Rates should have units of inverse time and will vary depending on the units of measurement of time; they can vary from 0 to infinity. However a number of terms, like *case-fatality rate, attack rate,* and *prevalence rate* are in widespread usage even though technically these are all proportions; i.e., they vary between 0 and 1 and are unitless.

10. The answer is C. *(Mausner, ed 2. pp 256–257.)* Net growth rate equals the birth rate minus the death rate plus the in-migration rate minus the out-migration rate; 17 − 10 + 2 = 9. Rates can be added or subtracted directly only if they are based on the same population denominator (in this case, the estimated midyear population).

11. The answer is E. *(Colton, pp 28–31.)* The correct values for mean, median, and mode are 3.4, 3, and 2. The *mean* is the average: the sum of the observations divided by the number of observations. In this case, the mean is 31 ÷ 9 = 3.4. The *median* is the middle observation in a series of ordered observations, i.e., the 50th percentile (when the number of observations is even, it is midway between the two middle observations). In this case, when the observations are ordered— 1,2,2,2,3,4,4,6,7—the median is 3. The *mode* is the observation that occurs with greatest frequency; in this case it is 2, which occurs three times.

12. The answer is D. *(Mausner, ed 2. pp 44–49.)* According to the table, 10 new cases of tuberculosis developed among the 500 individuals belonging to households with a case of tuberculosis at the time of the first survey. Because these 500 individuals were followed for 2 years, the number of person-years of exposure is 1,000. Therefore, the incidence rate is calculated as follows:

$$\frac{10 \text{ new cases}}{500 \text{ persons} \times 2 \text{ years}} = 10 \text{ cases per } 1,000 \text{ person-years}$$

(See also question 9.)

13. The answer is C. *(Mausner, ed 2. pp 44–49.)* Ten new cases of tuberculosis developed among 10,000 individuals belonging to households that had no culture-positive cases at the time of the first survey. Since these 10,000 individuals were followed for 2 years, the number of person-years of exposure is 20,000. Therefore the incidence rate is calculated as follows:

$$\frac{10 \text{ new cases}}{10,000 \text{ persons} \times 2 \text{ years}} = 0.5 \text{ cases per } 1,000 \text{ person-years}$$

14. The answer is E. *(Mausner, ed 2. p 169.)* The relative risk is the *ratio* of the incidence of a disease in a group exposed to a factor (in this case, household contact with tuberculosis) to the incidence in a group not exposed to the factor (persons without household contact.) Therefore, the relative risk is

$$\frac{\text{Incidence in households with exposure}}{\text{Incidence in households without exposure}} = \frac{10}{0.5} = 20$$

Identification of groups with a high level of relative risk can be useful in planning disease control programs.

15. The answer is D. *(Mausner, ed 2. pp 289–292.)* The identification of a specific factor (food) as a cause of illness (food poisoning) depends on comparing the proportion who became ill among those who did and those who did not eat each specified food (the proportion ill is sometimes called the "attack rate," but in fact it is a proportion, not a rate [see question 9]). The proportion ill among those who ate the food suspected of causing the disease should be significantly greater than among those who did not eat the food.

16. The answer is C. *(Colton, pp 115–119.)* The null hypothesis generally is that there is no difference between groups. The p value is the probability of obtaining a difference between groups at least as great as that observed in the study *if the null hypothesis were true*. Because it is calculated under the *assumption* that the null hypothesis is true, it cannot actually estimate the probability of the null hypothesis. If the p value is sufficiently high, the results are regarded as not statistically significant and the null hypothesis is not rejected. This, of course, does not mean that the two groups really are equivalent, only that the data did not provide sufficient evidence to conclude that they are different.

17. The answer is E. *(Mausner, ed 2. pp 155–156.)* In *experimental* studies, the investigators determine exposure of the study and control groups to a suspected causal factor and measure responses in the two groups. In *observational* studies, investigators have no control over exposure to a suspected causal factor but can measure responses in those who are and are not exposed. In both types of studies, the attempt is made to make the study and control groups similar in regard to all variables except exposure to the factor under study.

18. The answer is B. *(Schlesselman, pp 135–138.)* Misclassification bias, i.e., including people who do not really have the disease (controls) in the case groups, will tend to make the odds ratio falsely close to 1, rather than falsely high. (In the extreme example, where misclassification is so bad that both case and control groups are really equal mixtures of cases and controls, the odds ratio necessarily would equal 1.) Recall bias could cause a falsely high odds ratio; it is potentially a problem when using maternal recall to investigate exposures associated with birth defects. This study *is* a case-control study: the risk factor in this case is prenatal exposure to cigarette smoke. The placebo effect is of concern in unblinded intervention studies; it refers to the tendency of subjects to report improvement even when the treatment is not effective. It has no relevance to case-control studies.

19. The answer is B. *(Colton, pp 125–127.)* If the study described in the question is accurate, it suggests that baby boys whose mothers smoke are 2.6 times as likely to have undescended testes. This is because the odds ratio approximates the relative risk (risk ratio) unless the disease is very common. The fact that the 95 percent confidence interval excludes 1 means that $p < 0.05$. Confidence intervals describe the range of values not significantly different from the observed value, with a type 1 error rate (alpha) of 1 minus the level of confidence. Thus, a 95 percent confidence interval shows the numbers that are not statistically significantly different from what was observed at the 5 percent level. The lower the level of confidence, the narrower the confidence interval, so a 90 percent confidence interval would be narrower than a 95 percent confidence interval, in this case excluding 1.0 for certain.

20. The answer is B. *(Colton, pp 189–190.)* Because the goal of the study is to determine the correlation between serum levels of sodium and antidiuretic hormone (ADH) in patients who have meningitis, simultaneous determination of these paired variables in each member of a group of patients should be performed. The design described in choice A will allow only determination of the correlation within an individual or the variability of the assay methods; the design described in choice C will allow determination of the mean values of each variable but not their relationship; and the design described in choice D will permit comparison of ADH in cases and controls but will not provide data on serum levels of sodium.

21. The answer is D. *(Colton, pp 63–70.)* For two events or conditions, the probability that either will occur is the sum of their probabilities, minus the probability that both will occur. This is illustrated in the figure on the next page.

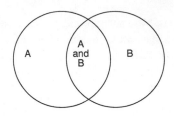

If we simply add the probability of A to the probability of B, the area labeled "A and B" will get counted twice. Therefore, the probability of (A and B) must be subtracted from the sum of the probabilities: p(A or B) = p(A) + p(B) − p(A and B). In this question, it is specifically stated that the two conditions are independent. When that is the case, the probability of both occurring is the product of their probabilities: p(A and B) = p(A) × p(B). The answer to this problem is 0.1 + 0.5 − (0.1)(0.5) = 0.55. Note that another common situation is when two conditions are mutually exclusive rather than independent (i.e., the probability of both occurring is zero). In this case, the probability of either one occurring is simply the sum of their probabilities. For example, if condition A were blue eyes, and condition B brown eyes, the probability of either blue or brown eyes would be 0.60.

22. The answer is D. *(Sackett, pp 127–131.)* Decision analysis begins with construction of a decision tree, i.e., outlining all possible outcomes, good and bad, of each decision. The next step involves estimation of the probabilities of these outcomes under each possible decision. The outcomes are then given ratings called *utilities*, which correspond to their relative desirability. The utilities and probabilities are then used together to compute the expected value of different decisions. Finally, in a process called *sensitivity analysis*, the probabilities and utilities are varied, to see how this affects the expected values of the different decisions. Calculation of sample size is not necessary for decision analysis because decision analysis is basically a pencil-and-paper (and computer) exercise: it does not require study subjects.

23. The answer is D. *(Ingelfinger, ed 2. pp 91–95.)* The normal (Gaussian) distribution is a symmetrical, bell-shaped distribution with many useful mathematical properties. Because it is symmetrical and unimodal, the mean is equal to the median and mode. It is entirely described by just two parameters: the mean and the standard deviation. The mean determines the location of the curve, the standard deviation how flat it is. As values get farther and farther from the mean, they become increasingly unlikely. Thus there are many more observations between 0 and 1 standard deviation from the mean than there are between 1 and 2 standard deviations from the mean.

24. The answer is B. *(Ingelfinger, ed 2. p 723.)* Sensitivity and specificity are measures of how often a diagnostic test gives the correct answer. Sensitivity reflects the test's performance in people who *have* the disease, and specificity measures the test's performance in people who *do not have* the disease. These definitions can be illustrated as follows:

	Disease Present	**Disease Absent**
Test +	True Positive (TP)	False Positive (FP)
Test −	False Negative (FN)	True Negative (TN)

Sensitivity = TP / (TP + FN)   Specificity = TN / (TN + FP)

Among people who have the disease, there are two possibilities: either the test correctly identifies them (TP), or it falsely classifies them as negative (FN). Thus among those with disease, sensitivity measures how often the test gives the right answer. (A good way to remember sensitivity is by the initials PID: positive in disease.) Similarly, among people who do not have the disease, there are also two possibilities: either the test will correctly identify them as not having disease (TN), or it will falsely classify them as diseased (FP). Thus specificity measures how often the test gives the right answer among those who do not have the disease. (A good way to remember specificity is by the initials NIH: negative in health.)

As opposed to sensitivity and specificity, which measure the test's performance in groups of patients who do and do not have the disease, *predictive value* measures how often the test is right in patients grouped another way: by whether the test result is positive or negative. Thus, predictive value of a positive test is the proportion of positive tests that are true positives [TP / (TP + FP)], and predictive value of a negative result is the proportion of negative test results that are true negatives [TN / (TN + FN)].

But predictive value is a little tricky because it also depends on the *prevalence* of the disease in the population tested. In this case, Dr. Stewells assembled groups of 100 patients with and without cholera, and the prevalence is not given. Therefore, predictive value cannot be calculated in this question, and the correct answer is B, since specificity is 88 percent, not 12 percent.

25. The answer is C. *(Ingelfinger, ed 2. pp 7–23.)* In this study of 1,000 patients with profuse diarrhea, 343 of them had cholera. Thus the prevalence of cholera (in this population) was 343/1,000. (Note that this is not an incidence because we are measuring existing cases, rather than new cases occurring over a period of time.) The predictive value of a positive result can thus be directly determined as TP/(TP + FP) = 312/(312 + 79) = 80 percent. Similarly, the predictive value of a negative result is TN/(TN + FN) = 578/(578 + 31) = 95 percent.

26. The answer is B. *(Ingelfinger, ed 2. pp 7–23.)* As the prevalence falls, more and more of those tested will *not* have cholera. This would not change either the sensitivity or specificity of the test, which do not depend on disease prevalence, but would affect predictive value: as prevalence falls, predictive value of a positive result also falls, whereas predictive value of a negative result rises. This makes sense: as a disease becomes more and more unlikely, positive test results should be viewed with increasing skepticism, whereas negative results become increasingly believable.

27. The answer is A. *(Colton, p 257.)* Randomization is the use of a predetermined plan of allocation or assignment of subjects to treatment groups such that assignment occurs solely by chance. It is used to eliminate bias on the part of the investigator and the subject in the choice of treatment group. The goal of randomization is to allow chance to distribute unknown sources of biological variability equally to the treatment and control groups. However, because chance does determine assignment, significant differences between the groups may arise, especially if the number of subjects is small. Therefore, whenever randomization is used, the comparability of the treatment groups should be assessed to determine whether or not balance was achieved.

28. The answer is D. *(Colton, pp 115–117.)* A p value of 0.60 indicates that the observed (or a greater) difference between the means could occur by chance as often as 6 times out of 10. This is not the same as saying that this result did occur by chance. Such a probability of chance is usually interpreted to mean that the result is not statistically significant. A value of p of 0.05 is the conventional upper limit of significance. However, even though p = 0.60, the null hypothesis of no difference between the means is not proved to be true. The most that can be said when the p value is not statistically significant is that the data are insufficient to cast doubt on the truth of the null hypothesis. If the samples were larger in size, the difference might be found to be statistically significant.

29. The answer is B. *(Mausner, ed 2. pp 156–159.)* The study described was a case-control study. In this type of study, people who have a disease (cases) are compared with people whom they closely resemble except for the presence of the disease under study (controls). Cases and controls are then studied for the frequency of exposure to a suspected risk factor. In case-control studies, the validity of inferences about the causal relationship between the exposure (cigarette smoking) and the disease (lung cancer) depends on how comparable the cases and controls are for all variables that may be related to both the risk factor and disease under study (e.g., age, sex, race, place of residence, and occupation).

30. The answer is E. *(Mausner, ed 2. pp 344–345.)* The most important risk factor for breast cancer (like most cancers) is age: the rate in women 75 to 84 years old is about 50 times that of women 35 to 44 years old. If crude incidence rates are compared (new cases per 100,000 adult women), one country may have much larger numbers of women in the peak risk groups and have a much higher incidence for that reason. Therefore, either comparison of the age-specific rates for each age group, or else some type of *age adjustment* is essential. Although nursing may have a protective effect on breast cancer, it is of nowhere near the magnitude of the effect of age. Cigarette smoke is not a major risk factor for breast cancer. Early diagnosis, if it had any effect, would be expected to increase the incidence rate (since some cases might be discovered that otherwise might spontaneously resolve or not be noticed before the woman died of another cause). Finally, efficacy of treatment might affect the death rate, but would not affect the incidence of the disease.

31–33. The answers are: 31-D, 32-B, 33-E. *(Rothman, pp 311–313.)* The *excess risk* is the incidence in those exposed to the risk factors minus the incidence in those unexposed. Thus, the excess risk from drinking among nonsmokers is $30 - 10 = 20$ cases per 10,000 person-years. Similarly, for smoking (among nondrinkers) it is $50 - 10 = 40$ cases per 10,000 person-years. The *relative risk* for smoking among nondrinkers is $50 / 10 = 5.0$, but the overall relative risk also depends on the relative risk in drinkers, which may be higher, lower, or the same. The overall relative risk also depends on the proportion of the population that drinks: the lower that proportion, the closer the overall relative risk will be to that of nondrinkers. To determine which risk factor is the cause of a greater number of cases (*population attributable fraction,* sometimes called *attributable risk*) requires knowledge of the prevalence of the risk factor, as well as its relative risk.

When there is more than one risk factor for a disease, it is important to compare the risk in those with both risk factors with that expected under different models of causation. Under an additive model, when risk factors are independent, *excess risks add.* Thus the excess risk for smoking and drinking would be $20 + 40 = 60$. To give an excess risk of 60 requires that $X = 70$.

Under a multiplicative model, when risk factors are independent, *relative risks multiply.* Thus the relative risk for patients with both risk factors should be $3 \times 5 = 15$. Thus X must be $15 \times 10 = 150$.

These questions demonstrate that determining the presence of independence, synergy, or antagonism among risk factors requires clear specification of whether one is dealing with an additive or multiplicative model of causation.

34. The answer is E (all). *(Mausner, ed 2. pp 185–186.)* When the suspected causal factor cannot be manipulated by the researcher for ethical or practical reasons (e.g., exposure of pregnant women to rubella), observational studies must be performed to determine whether observed associations are causally related. The judgment of causality is based on several types of evidence:

a. Strength of the association. Chance is an important basis for observed associations that must be ruled out. Low p values make chance a less likely explanation for an association.

b. Consistency in different studies. This is the reproducibility of observations on the basis of the scientific method. Replication of the observed association in different populations in independent studies strengthens the judgment of causality.

c. Time sequence. The two factors must occur in the proper sequence in which the putative cause precedes the putative effect.

d. Consistency with existing knowledge (biologic plausibility). The observations should be consistent or compatible with existing biological knowledge.

35. The answer is D (4). *(Mausner, ed 2. pp 43–45.)* Neither incidence nor prevalence of leukemia can be determined from the data given in the table without knowledge of the population at risk for leukemia and served by the study hospital. The data given provide numerators, but the lack of age-specific data on population prevents calculation of rates. The only conclusion (among those given in the question) that can be based on the data is that in the period 1970 to 1984 the number of children admitted to the hospital with a diagnosis of leukemia increased for the 0 to 9 age group.

36. The answer is C (2, 4). *(Lilienfeld, ed 2. pp 217–218.)* The attributable risk estimates the importance of a particular risk factor as a cause of the disease. The importance depends on the prevalence of the risk factor because if hardly anyone in the population has the risk factor, it is unlikely to explain very many cases of the disease. The importance of a risk factor also depends on how strong a risk factor it is, as measured by the relative risk. The formula for calculating attributable risk is

$$\frac{p(RR - 1)}{p(RR - 1) + 1}$$

where p is the prevalence of the risk factor in the population, and RR is the relative risk of the disease for the risk factor. For smoking, p is about 0.3, and RR about 20, giving an attributable risk of about 85 percent. Note that the term *attributable risk* is defined differently by different authors, so that it is helpful to specify exactly what is meant when the term is used. Synonyms for the definition supplied here are *population attributable fraction* and *etiologic fraction*.

37. The answer is C (2, 4). *(Colton, pp 100–107, 115–116, 124.)* The p value depends not only on the magnitude of the difference between groups (larger differences leading to smaller p values), but also on the sample size of the study. For a true difference of a given size, the p value can be made as small as desired by increasing the sample size. However, if there really is no difference between the groups (i.e., if the null hypothesis is true), the chance of obtaining statistical significance at the 0.05 level will always be 0.05, regardless of the size of the sample.

The standard error of the mean (SEM) is sometimes confused with the standard deviation (SD). Whereas the SD is a measure of dispersion of individual measurements about the mean, the SEM is a measure of variation of sample means about the population mean (see question 3). The "tails" in a significance test refer to the tails of the statistical distributions used to calculate the p values. A one-tailed test is the less conservative; i.e., it more often leads to rejection of the null hypothesis when it is true. Just remember: if you double the number of tails, you double the p value.

38. The answer is D (4). *(Ingelfinger, ed 2. pp 258–263.)* As a general rule, it is much easier to get a falsely negative result on a randomized blinded trial than a falsely positive result. The reason is that errors will tend to affect both treatment groups, making it harder to show a difference between them. Thus in this question, inclusion of subjects without the ear effusion (who could not benefit from the intervention) and incorrect determination of which effusions resolved would both lead to falsely negative, not falsely positive results. Similarly, a small sample size is a reason for a falsely negative, but not a falsely positive result. Only chance (random error) or a breakdown in the blinding or randomization process would be causes of a falsely positive result.

39. The answer is E (all). *(Mausner, ed 2. pp 200, 348–352.)* Sample size for a clinical trial depends on the frequency with which the outcome occurs in the control group, the magnitude of the effect that is to be detected, and the type 1 and type 2 error rates, alpha and beta. (A type 1 error occurs when the study erroneously finds a difference between two groups; a type 2 error is when the two groups really are different, but the study does not reach that conclusion.) An additional consideration in prospective studies, particularly those of long duration, is loss to follow-up, including mortality from causes not under investigation.

40. The answer is E (all). *(National Center for Health Statistics, pp 3, 48–60, 65.)* The 1978 revision of the U.S. Standard Report of Fetal Death is recommended for state-wide adoption by the National Center for Health Statistics and is designed to collect information that includes the cause of fetal death, demographic data, complications and duration of pregnancy, the weight of the fetus, the characteristics of prenatal care, and labor complications. Some states, because of differing definitions of fetal death, require a fetal death certificate only in cases where gestation has reached the twentieth week; other states require a certificate for all products of conception. While a physician is required to indicate whether an autopsy was performed and, if so, whether the results were used to determine the cause of death, the actual results of an autopsy are not required. In fact, usually a death certificate must be completed by the physician long before autopsy results are available. The weight of the fetus is considered by the Public Health Service to be the primary parameter to allow evaluation of fetal viability.

41. The answer is E (all). *(Mausner, ed 2. pp 180–183.)* The statistical significance of any association between variables merely is an assessment of the probability of observing such an association by chance. Even with a statistical significance of p = 0.01, one in a hundred times such an association would be expected to occur owing to chance. If chance is unlikely, the association could be artifactual (owing to bias in the study design), indirect (because the factors under study are related to each other as the result of some common associated or intervening factor), or causal.

42. The answer is D (4). *(Ingelfinger, ed 2. pp 190–197.)* The finding of a statistically significant association on linear regression analysis does not prove that an association is linear, nor that it is causal, nor that it is large or important. Exponential, logarithmic, quadratic, threshold, and many other associations can lead to statistically significant linear regression coefficients. Choice 2 is incorrect because it implies causality, which was not demonstrated. To be able to say that lead and IQ were *independently* associated requires knowledge that other potentially confounding variables (e.g., social class) were controlled for, as with multiple linear regression.

43. The answer is C (2, 4). *(Wegman, Pediatrics 80:817–827, 1987.)* Infant mortality is defined as the number of deaths in infants up to 1 year of age per 1,000 live births. It is further divided into neonatal mortality, which includes deaths up to 28 days of age, and postneonatal mortality, which includes deaths from 28 days to 1 year of age. In the U.S., about two-thirds of infant mortality occurs in the first 28 days of life, and the most important cause is prematurity. The most important cause of postneonatal mortality is the sudden infant death syndrome (SIDS). American blacks have twice the rates of low birth weight, neonatal mortality, and postneonatal mortality of whites.

44. The answer is E (all). *(Hulley, pp 78–86.)* Controls are an integral part of a case-control study. They provide a means of evaluating whether the frequency (or level) of a characteristic (or past event) among persons with the disease (the cases) is different from that in comparable persons in the population who do not have the condition being investigated (the controls). The choice of cases in a case-control study is often straightforward: all available and accessible cases may need to be studied. On the other hand, a major challenge of case-control studies is selection of the controls, a process that involves some balancing of scientific validity against cost and inconvenience.

45. The answer is A (1, 2, 3). *(Mausner, ed 2. pp 155, 312–316.)* In cohort studies, a group of subjects is defined on the basis of certain baseline characteristics and followed over time for the development of the disease (or other outcome) under study. The incidence of disease in subjects with various characteristics can then be compared with the incidence in subjects without those characteristics. Because cohort studies are used to test specific hypotheses, they are *analytic*, rather than *descriptive*.

46. The answer is D (4). *(Ingelfinger, ed 2. pp 8–9.)* The choice of an optimal cutoff for a screening test often involves weighing the relative benefits of sensitivity and specificity. There is no set rule about which is the more important; rather, the decision must depend upon the consequences of false positive or false negative results. For example, because there is no good treatment for amyotrophic lateral sclerosis, a delay in diagnosis (or a missed diagnosis) caused by an insensitive test would be of little consequence. But since the diagnosis of ALS could end the search for a treatable cause of the patient's symptoms, a false positive result could be devastating. Thus for ALS, specificity is far more important than sensitivity. The situation is reversed for neonatal hypothyroidism, in which consequences of a false negative test (i.e., a child with hypothyroidism is missed by the test) are much worse than consequences of a false positive test (additional tests or even unnecessary thyroid hormone).

47. The answer is A (1, 2, 3). *(Colton, pp 136–139.)* The student t test for the comparison of two means rests on the following assumptions: independence of the samples, and equal standard deviations and normal distributions of the variable in the two populations being sampled. The mathematical basis of the t test assumes that the distributions of the samples are approximately normal; however, the samples do not have to be equal in size.

48–51. The answers are: 48-B, 49-A, 50-C, 51-D. *(Colton, pp 40–41, 131–133, 137–139, 174–177.)* Use of the student t test to assess the difference between the mean systolic pressures of pregnant and nonpregnant women would be appropriate since the two groups are independent samples and the outcome variable is quantitative and approximately normally distributed.

In the study comparing the occurrence of hepatitis B surface antigen in medical and dental students, use of chi-square analysis would be appropriate because both the predictor and outcome variables are dichotomous; that is, students are classified by the presence or absence of the antigen and by medical or dental student status.

To compare the levels of blood glucose in rats to whom a drug was administered, analysis of variance would be appropriate because six different groups are to be analyzed (two sexes and three drugs). Analysis of variance will permit evaluation of the effects and interaction of sex and drug on the glucose level.

The paired t test is appropriate for comparing paired (e.g., before and after) measurements. Use of the regular (student two-sample) t test in this instance is incorrect, because the two samples are not independent—the same subjects are in each.

52–55. The answers are: 52-A, 53-C, 54-B, 55-E. *(Mausner, ed 2. pp 47, 49, 55–56, 149–152, 312, 317.)* The *point prevalence* is the proportion of people in a population who have a disease at a given point in time. The numerator is the number of existing cases of a disease; the denominator is the total population at risk of the disease at that point in time.

In order to compare rates of disease or death in two or more groups that differ substantially in age, sex, or racial structure, adjustment or standardization of the rates is necessary to remove the effects of those differences. The *standardized mortality or morbidity ratio* (SMR) is the ratio of the observed number to the expected number of deaths or cases of the disease. For example, age-specific rates of angina pectoris in nonsmokers can be applied to the age distribution of smokers to obtain the expected number of cases of angina pectoris in the smokers. The SMR of smokers for angina pectoris is the observed number of cases divided by the expected number so calculated.

The *incidence rate* is the number of new cases of a disease that occur in a period of time divided by the population at risk during that time.

The *relative risk* is the incidence of disease in subjects with a risk factor divided by the incidence in those in whom the factor is absent. (The denominator is *not* the incidence in the general population, since subjects *with* the risk factor would be included.) The term *relative risk* can be confusing when the risk factor has to do with being a *relative* of a patient; in this instance *risk ratio* is a preferable synonym.

56–59. The answers are: 56-B, 57-E, 58-A, 59-C. *(Mausner, ed 2. pp 54–55, 264, 280–281.)* The *case-fatality rate* is a measure of the severity of a disease. It is a ratio of the number of deaths caused by a disease to the total number of cases of that disease and is usually expressed as a percentage. The *crude mortality* equals the total number of deaths from all causes during a year divided by the average population at risk during that year. It is usually expressed as the number of deaths per 1,000 people. The *secondary attack rate* is a measure of the contagiousness of an infectious disease. The numerator is the number of cases of disease occurring in contacts of the index case; the denominator is the number of contacts exposed to the index case during a specified period. Rates of disease are called *morbidity rates*.

60–63. The answers are: 60-A, 61-B, 62-B, 63-A. *(Ehrlich, Pediatrics 70:665, 1982. Siegel, pp 315–344.)* One of the most commonly made statistical errors is use of tests that assume that each of the observations is independent on data sets that violate that assumption. Be very suspicious that this assumption might be violated any time the denominators are greater than the number of study subjects. For example, in question 60, even though group sizes were 24 and 9, denominators for the proportions compared were 231 and 55. If observations are independent, it means that each observation gives the same amount of information. For dichotomous (yes/no) variables, as in this example, it means that the probability of a ''yes'' is the same for each observation. Returning to the example of urine cultures, since the overall proportion of positive cultures was 34/55 in the diversion group, it means that the best estimate of the probability that each culture will be positive should be 34/55. But what if one particular patient had received 20 of those cultures, and 19 had been positive? The best estimate of the probability that another culture from that person would be positive is 19/20, not 34/55. Thus if one wishes to estimate the probability of a positive culture in an individual, not all the observations in the sample give the same amount of information: previous cultures on the same person would be more informative than cultures on others.

The situation is similar (though a bit more subtle) in question 63. Here the denominators are (appropriately) children, but once again, not all observations are independent. The trouble here is that all the subjects are in four classrooms, and if one child in the class develops chickenpox, other children in that class are much more likely to do so. For example, if by chance the one new contact with chickenpox happened to be in one of the control group classes, many people in that class would be infected. As was the case with urine cultures, if one wanted to estimate the probability that a specific child would get chickenpox, not all observations would be equally informative: observations on other members of the same class would be much more relevant.

Another very commonly made error is use of statistics that assume that the data are normally distributed when that assumption is false. This is the error in questions 61 and 62. The normal distribution is bell-shaped, symmetrical, and continuous. Data with a limited number of categories (such as parity) violate the assumption of normality, particularly if the mode is not somewhere near the middle category. The other main way in which the normality assumption is violated is by very skewed distributions, i.e., asymmetric distributions that have some very extreme values on one side. Length of hospital stay is a good example: A single patient with a very complicated hospital course may tremendously affect the mean length of stay, and its standard deviation in whichever group that patient is in. (Note that to some extent, these two effects cancel each other out because they tend to affect the p value in opposite directions. The statistical way of saying this is that the t test is fairly *robust* to violations of the assumption of normality.) A helpful rule is this: There should be equal numbers of values at the mean plus and minus two standard deviations. In questions 61 and 62, values of < 1.0 or 1.5 standard deviations below the mean were not possible: a negative length of stay or a negative number of children would result because in each case the mean is less than 2.0 standard deviations from a lower limit for the variable. Whenever the assumption of normality is not reasonable, the data should be analyzed using a nonparametric technique, such as a rank sum test. In the example regarding length of hospital stay, it is quite possible that use of a nonparametric technique would lead to a lower p value, if, for example, there was one patient in the medical group with a very long length of stay.

64–67. The answers are: 64-D, 65-A, 66-B, 67-D. *(Colton, pp 6–7, 243–244.)* For proper comparison of the frequency of a disease in two groups, the rate of disease, not the number of cases, must be compared. The number of cases may reflect the age structure of the population served by the hospital. Age-specific attack rates that incorporate the number of cases in each age group, divided by the number of persons in each group, should be calculated.

In order to determine that an association between two conditions such as diabetes and obesity exists, an investigator must show that obesity is significantly more common in persons who have diabetes than in persons who do not have diabetes. The controls are necessary in order to test the significance of the association and must resemble the cases as closely as possible in all ways except for the absence of the disease under study.

Whenever considerable numbers of a cohort are lost to follow-up, doubts about the validity of the conclusions arise. Because death may be a major reason for loss to follow-up, the most conservative approach is to assume that everyone lost to follow-up has died. Unless, in this example, the death rate in the anxiety neurosis cohort was *still* no greater than that in the general population (after adding another 50 deaths for the 20 percent of the 250 patients lost to follow-up), the conclusions are suspect.

The conclusion in question 67 is invalid because of the lack of denominators to calculate the rate of bacterial endocarditis in different age groups. In addition, the autopsy series merely gives an estimate of the proportion of deaths in different age groups, not the frequency of occurrence of endocarditis with age. The autopsy series may also be invalid as a source of data from which to draw conclusions because of factors that determined whether an autopsy was performed.

68–71. The answers are: 68-B, 69-A, 70-E, 71-B. *(Hulley, pp 99–108. Mausner, ed 2. pp 329–332.)* Matching is a way of selecting subjects that are comparable with respect to specific variables. For example, in a case-control study, a control could be selected that is the same age and sex as the case. It is thus a *sampling* strategy to achieve comparability among groups.

Stratification is an analysis strategy with the same purpose. Thus, after the study has been completed, the subjects can be stratified, i.e., divided into separate, relatively homogeneous strata, and the comparison between groups can occur within each stratum. For example, survival could be compared separately in different age strata, as in question 68. This might be important if the subjects with high renin levels were also older than the subjects with low levels, since a difference in survival between the two groups might be due to age, rather than to differing renin levels.

Age adjustment takes stratification by age one step further. After mortality (or another parameter) is calculated for specific age strata, it is combined in a weighted average to yield a single number. The weights used are the sizes of the different age strata in a standard population. Age adjustment is used most often for comparing mortality in populations with differing age structures.

Multivariate statistical analysis, like stratification, is an analysis technique for achieving comparability among groups. It involves *modeling* the associations between variables in order to allow their different effects to be isolated from each other. (For example, in multiple regression, the relationships between variables are modeled as a straight line.)

Survival analysis is a technique by which persons followed for variable lengths of time are counted according to the length of time they were followed. For example, in the cohort study of renin levels mentioned above, instead of simply comparing the proportions surviving 5 years, the cumulative probability of survival could be plotted for the two groups, and the two curves compared.

72–75. The answers are: 72-A, 73-D, 74-E, 75-C. *(Hulley, pp 204–205.)* If the probability of an event is p, the *odds* of the event are $p/(1 - p)$. The *odds ratio* is the ratio of the odds of exposure to the risk factor given disease (a/c) to the odds of exposure to the risk factor given no disease (b/d). To illustrate that the odds of exposure given disease are a/c, the probability of exposure given disease is $p = a/(a + c)$. So $(1 - p) = c/(a + c)$, and the odds are $[a/(a + c)]/[c/(a + c)]$, and the $(a + c)$'s cancel out to give a/c. The odds ratio, therefore, is (a/c)/(b/d), which equals ad/bc.

Odds ratios are mainly used in case-control studies, from which relative risk cannot be calculated directly. When the disease is rare, the odds ratio closely approximates the relative risk. However, the study in the example is a cohort study, so relative risk can be calculated directly from the table. It is equal to the risk (incidence) of suicide in those who served in Vietnam divided by the risk in those who served elsewhere, or $[a/(a + b)]/[c/(c + d)]$.

Excess risk is defined as the *difference* between the risk in those with the risk factor and those in whom it is absent. Whereas the relative risk and odds ratio are unitless (since any measurement of time in the denominators cancels out), the excess risk must have an explicit or implied time period on the denominator. In this example, $a/(a + b) - c/(c + d)$ represents the excess risk of suicide in Vietnam veterans over a 5-year period; it is five times as big as the excess risk for a 1-year period. Thus, if the yearly risk of suicide was 0.2 percent in Vietnam veterans and 0.1 percent in other veterans, the relative risk would be 2.0, and the excess risk (risk difference) 0.1 percent per year, or 0.5 percent over the 5-year period.

The overall incidence of suicide (per 5 years) in the study is simply the number of suicides (a + c) divided by the population at risk (a + b + c + d). (Note that a more precise way to measure the incidence, relative risk, and so on would be to use person-years at risk on the denominators, but this leads to greater computational and conceptual complexity.)

76–79. The answers are: 76-C, 77-E, 78-A, 79-D. *(Hulley, pp 24–25.)* Simple *random sampling* is a process in which individuals are sampled independently, and each individual of the population has an equal probability of being selected.

In *cluster sampling,* groups of people (e.g., families, school classes) are selected at random, and then everyone in those groups is sampled. A common analytic mistake is to pretend that subjects obtained in a cluster sample were obtained in a simple random sample. This can lead to incorrect results, because the subjects are not really independent of each other.

Systematic sampling is a process that first requires the arrangement of the group to be sampled in some kind of order. Then individuals are selected systematically throughout the series on the basis of a predetermined sampling fraction or constant determinant, for example, every fifth, tenth, or hundredth person in the ordered group. Although systematic sampling may seem almost the same as simple random sampling, it is much less desirable. For example, sampling every other subject from a list in which husbands' and wives' names appear next to each other (e.g., an alphabetical list) will bias the sample—if husbands were always first, the sample might include no wives and would rarely include both persons in a married couple.

By *stratified sampling,* a population is divided into subgroups based on defined characteristics such as age, sex, or severity of illness, or any combination of these; then random samples are selected from each subgroup.

In *paired sampling,* or *matching,* selection of one or more controls for each case is based on age, sex, time, time sequence, geographic location, or some other defined relationship to the case. For example, selection could be based on the next patient admitted after each case, the nearest-age sibling to each case, or the person who lives closest geographically to each case.

80–82. The answers are: 80-D, 81-B, 82-C. *(Mausner, ed 2. pp 78–79, 85–87.)* Meningococcal meningitis, because of its severity and the fear of epidemics, is reportable in all states. Reporting of meningococcal meningitis to local and state health departments by physicians tends to be more complete than reporting of less severe diseases such as measles, German measles, or salmonellosis. Many states improve the completeness of their infectious disease surveillance by requiring all diagnostic laboratories to report the isolation of certain pathogenic microbes.

The incidence and prevalence of chronic diseases such as arthritis are difficult to determine because patients who have arthritis often do not need hospitalization. The National Health Interview Survey uses data obtained by conducting household surveys of defined populations and attempts continuously to provide data on the health status and needs of the country.

In several states and foreign countries, all newly diagnosed cases of cancer occurring in a defined geographic area are reported to a cancer registry and then followed by the registry until death of the patients. Such registries provide very important information on the incidence, prevalence, and survival rates of different types of cancers. In addition, the registries provide a source of cases for case-control studies and other research.

83–86. The answers are: 83-B, 84-D, 85-A, 86-E. *(Colton, pp 28–31.)* Mean, median, and mode are all measures of central tendency, while variance, standard deviation, and range are measures of dispersion. In figure B, both distributions appear normally shaped, and they center on the same point, but curve 2 has greater variance because it is more spread out. Figure D, in contrast, shows two distributions with the same variance, but different means. In figure A, both the centers and the shapes of the curves differ. Curve one is skewed to the right, which means it has more of a tail on the right side.

Remember that the value that occurs most commonly (i.e., the highest point on the curve) is the mode, so choice E represents "pi a la mode"—a very tasty dessert.

87–90. The answers are: 87-C, 88-A, 89-B, 90-D. *(Browner, JAMA 257:2459–2463, 1987. Michael, pp 31–38, 91–95, 105–112.)* A type 2 error occurs when a study fails to reject the null hypothesis (of no effect), when it is in fact false. Any time a study fails to achieve statistical significance, a crucial question to ask is whether the study had enough subjects. Although 500 subjects per group followed for 5 years seems like a larger number, only a tiny minority (perhaps 10 per group) would be expected to have a myocardial infarction. Thus the sample size in this instance may have been inadequate to detect a meaningful difference between the groups.

The ecologic fallacy occurs when associations among groups of subjects are mistakenly assumed to hold for individuals. Thus although among communities high rates of condom use may be associated with higher fertility rates (perhaps because condom use acts as a marker for sexual activity in general), among those who use the condoms, the fertility rate could in fact be zero.

A type 1 error occurs when, just by chance, a statistically significant difference between groups is found. Studies attempting to correlate multiple risk factors with multiple diseases (particularly when there is no good biological reason to suspect an association) are especially prone to type 1 errors.

Selection bias occurs when the subjects selected for the study are somehow not representative of the population from which they come. One trouble with selecting spouses for controls is that one's spouse is much more likely to share one's smoking habits than a person from the general population. Thus, since patients with lung cancer will be mostly smokers, smokers will be overrepresented among the controls, and smoking will look like a weaker risk factor than it really is.

91–95. The answers are: 91-A, 92-C, 93-E, 94-B, 95-D. *(Last, ed 2. p 80.)* The scale of measurement is an important determinant of the amount of information in a variable, and the type of statistical analysis that can be used. Dichotomous variables (like sex) have only two possible values. Some variables may be artificially dichotomized, with subsequent loss of information. For example, a patient either survives 5 years or not; thus survival to 5 years is an example of a dichotomous variable. The variable could be made more informative, however, if the actual number of months of survival was specified.

Nominal variables have more than two possible values, but no intrinsic ordering. Race is the classic example; medical specialties also have no intrinsic ordering. Nominal and ordinal are often confused. Just remember *no*minal for *no* ordering.

Ordinal variables are intrinsically ordered, but not in a quantitative way that allows one to say that there is a natural numerical distance between possible values.

Thus one value cannot really be subtracted from another. Examples are qualitative judgments like "worse, same, better" or "never, sometimes, always." Remember, *ord*inal means *ord*ered.

Interval scales are ordered, but with real numerical units; they can be subtracted from each other. An example is dates of birth: they are intrinsically ordered, and subtracting them gives meaningful numbers, but there is no intrinsic zero to the scale, so that dividing them does not make a lot of sense—one birthdate cannot be twice as big as another.

Ratio scales are measurements in relation to a clear zero point. Thus measurements on ratio scales can be meaningfully divided by each other. For example, one baby may weigh twice as much as another, or have twice as high a platelet count. Absolute temperature is measured on a ratio scale, whereas temperature in Fahrenheit or Celsius is measured on an interval scale.

Communicable Diseases

DIRECTIONS: Each question below contains five suggested responses. Select the **one best** response to each question.

96. Which of the following is the most common cause of intrauterine infection of the fetus in the United States?

(A) Rubella
(B) Syphilis
(C) Cytomegalovirus
(D) Toxoplasmosis
(E) Herpes simplex

97. The incidence of nosocomial infections among patients admitted to general hospitals in the United States is about

(A) 1 percent
(B) 3 percent
(C) 6 percent
(D) 12 percent
(E) 18 percent

98. Which of the following statements regarding herpes simplex virus, type 2 (HSV-2), is correct?

(A) Infections with HSV-2 are almost always symptomatic
(B) Transmission from mother to infant is generally transplacental
(C) HSV infection is an early sign of the acquired immunodeficiency syndrome
(D) Neonates with cutaneous disease should receive antiviral therapy regardless of whether there is evidence of dissemination
(E) None of the above

99. The occurrence of a group of illnesses of similar nature at a rate above the expected number is called

(A) hyperendemic
(B) epidemic
(C) endemic
(D) enzootic
(E) pandemic

100. Chickenpox is associated with

(A) a high case fatality rate
(B) congenital malformations in 10 percent of offspring of infected mothers
(C) a high reinfection rate
(D) a long prodromal period
(E) Reye syndrome

101. The time interval between entry of an infectious agent into a host and the onset of symptoms is called

(A) the communicable period
(B) the incubation period
(C) the preinfectious period
(D) the noncontagious period
(E) none of the above

102. The newborn with cytomegalovirus infection at birth most commonly presents with

(A) hepatosplenomegaly
(B) hepatitis
(C) thrombocytopenia
(D) cerebral calcifications
(E) no symptoms

103. Immunization of preschool children with diphtheria toxoid results in

(A) protection against the diphtheria carrier state
(B) lifelong immunity against diphtheria
(C) detectable antitoxin for about 10 years
(D) frequent adverse reactions
(E) protection against infection of the respiratory tract by *Corynebacterium diphtheriae*

104. Epidemics of typhus fever have been associated with war and famine for several centuries. What factor was most important in the control of such epidemics following the end of World War II?

(A) Eradication of *Anopheles* mosquitoes
(B) Improved sanitation practices
(C) Improved methods for handling food supplies
(D) Disinfestation by use of DDT
(E) Mass therapy with antibiotics

Questions 105–107

In a study of the effectiveness of pertussis vaccine in preventing pertussis (whooping cough), the following data were collected by studying siblings of children who had the disease.

Immunization Status of Sibling Contact	Number of Siblings Exposed to Case	Number of Cases among Siblings
Complete	4,000	400
None	1,000	400

105. What was the secondary attack rate of pertussis in fully immunized household contacts?

(A) 0 percent
(B) 10 percent
(C) 25 percent
(D) 40 percent
(E) 75 percent

106. What was the protective efficacy of whooping cough vaccine?

(A) 25 percent
(B) 40 percent
(C) 75 percent
(D) 90 percent
(E) None of the above

107. What was the relative risk of contacting whooping cough in the un-immunized children compared with the fully immunized children?

(A) 0.25
(B) 0.5
(C) 1.0
(D) 2.0
(E) 4.0

Questions 108–110

Data from an investigation of an epidemic of German measles in a remote village in Brazil are given in the table below:

Age Group (in years)	Number in Population	Number Ill (symptomatic)	Number Not Ill but with Antibody Rise (asymptomatic)	Number Uninfected	Percent Infected
0–9	204	110	74	20	90
10–19	129	70	46	13	90
20–39	161	88	57	16	90
40–59	78	42	28	8	90
60+	42	2	2	38	10
Totals	614	312	207	95	

108. Which expression represents the calculation to determine the incidence of illness for all age groups (as a percentage)?

(A) $\dfrac{312}{614} \times 100\% = 50.8\%$

(B) $\dfrac{207}{614} \times 100\% = 33.7\%$

(C) $\dfrac{95}{519} \times 100\% = 18.3\%$

(D) $\dfrac{519}{614} \times 100\% = 84.5\%$

(E) $\dfrac{207}{519} \times 100\% = 39.9\%$

109. Which expression represents the calculation to determine the percentage of infection that is asymptomatic (subclinical)?

(A) $\dfrac{312}{614} \times 100\% = 50.8\%$

(B) $\dfrac{207}{614} \times 100\% = 33.7\%$

(C) $\dfrac{95}{519} \times 100\% = 18.3\%$

(D) $\dfrac{519}{614} \times 100\% = 84.5\%$

(E) $\dfrac{207}{519} \times 100\% = 39.9\%$

110. Based on the age-specific infection rates, approximately when did German measles previously occur in this village—in relation to the current epidemic?

(A) 1 to 9 years ago
(B) 10 to 19 years ago
(C) 20 to 39 years ago
(D) 40 to 59 years ago
(E) 60 years ago

111. The administration of a single injection of live attenuated measles vaccine results in

(A) seroconversion in 95 percent of susceptible children
(B) the induction of active immunity that lasts less than 5 years
(C) postimmunization encephalitis in 0.1 percent of recipients
(D) subacute sclerosing panencephalitis in 0.017 percent of recipients
(E) no significant risk to children with leukemia

112. Which of the following bacteria is the most common cause of bacterial meningitis in children 3 months to 6 years of age in the United States?

(A) *Streptococcus pneumoniae*
(B) *Neisseria meningitidis*
(C) *Haemophilus influenzae* type b
(D) *Escherichia coli* K1
(E) Group B *Streptococcus hemolyticus*

113. Which of the following statements concerning the ELISA test for the presence of antibodies to the human immunodeficiency virus (HIV; the AIDS virus) is true?

(A) Only about 10 percent of those with antibodies to the virus (i.e., a true positive ELISA test) will get AIDS
(B) The presence of antibody correlates well with protective immunity
(C) The ELISA test has a low positive predictive value when low-risk populations are screened
(D) False positive tests sometimes occur in patients with far-advanced AIDS
(E) People whose ELISA test is negative cannot transmit HIV to others

114. The bacteria that are involved in nosocomial (hospital-associated) infections are transmitted most often by

(A) airborne matter
(B) fomites
(C) exposure to a common source
(D) indwelling catheters
(E) direct contact via hands

115. Which is the most common site of hospital-acquired infections?

(A) Surgical wound
(B) Respiratory tract
(C) Skin
(D) Urinary tract
(E) Gastrointestinal tract

116. All the following statements about diphtheria, pertussis, and tetanus are true EXCEPT

(A) immunization against the three diseases should be begun at 2 months of age
(B) most adults are not immune to pertussis
(C) the pertussis vaccine is a toxoid that is relatively frequently associated with adverse effects
(D) tetanus immune globulin should be given for dirty wounds only if the patient's tetanus immunizations are not up to date
(E) adults should receive a diphtheria booster at the time of their tetanus boosters (as a dT)

117. Which of the following statements concerning skin testing for tuberculosis is correct?

(A) All children should be tested yearly with intermediate-strength purified protein derivative (PPD)
(B) Children with positive tests do not require treatment if their chest x-ray is negative
(C) Compared with children, adults with tuberculosis are much less likely to be contagious
(D) Atypical mycobacteria may cause false positive results
(E) None of the above

118. Which of the following statements about *Giardia lamblia,* the cause of giardiasis, is correct?

(A) The primary site of infection is the colon
(B) Liver involvement is rare, except in immunosuppressed patients
(C) Bloody diarrhea, cramps, and fever are seen in severe cases
(D) The incubation period is 1 to 3 days
(E) None of the above

DIRECTIONS: Each question below contains four suggested responses of which **one or more** is correct. Select

A	if	**1, 2, and 3**	are correct
B	if	**1 and 3**	are correct
C	if	**2 and 4**	are correct
D	if	**4**	is correct
E	if	**1, 2, 3, and 4**	are correct

119. Preventive treatment with isoniazid (isonicotinic acid hydrazide) is recommended for which of the following groups?

(1) Young adults in whom a positive tuberculin test is demonstrated
(2) Children under age 3 in whom a positive tuberculin test is demonstrated
(3) All members of a household in which one member has an active case of tuberculosis
(4) Children with atypical mycobacterial infection

120. True statements about Lyme disease include

(1) it is caused by an arthropod-borne virus (arbovirus)
(2) it is associated with a characteristic skin rash, called erythema marginatum centrificum (EMC)
(3) it occurs primarily in the Rocky Mountain states of the U.S.
(4) it may involve the heart and the central nervous system, as well as joints

121. True statements regarding type B *Haemophilus influenzae* include that

(1) it is a more important cause of mortality in children than in adults
(2) polysaccharide vaccine conjugated with diphtheria toxoid should be given to children at 18 months of age
(3) it is the major cause of acute epiglottitis
(4) it is the most common cause of acute otitis media in children

122. Reasons to treat gonorrhea with tetracycline 500 mg p.o. q.i.d. for 7 days, rather than with ampicillin 3.5 g p.o. plus probenecid 1 g p.o. taken at one time, include

(1) lower frequency of side effects
(2) greater safety in case of pregnancy
(3) enhanced compliance
(4) better coverage of *Chlamydia trachomatis*

SUMMARY OF DIRECTIONS

A	B	C	D	E
1,2,3 only	1,3 only	2,4 only	4 only	All are correct

123. Effective means of preventing trichinosis in humans include

(1) cooking pork and pork products to ensure that all parts of the meat reach a temperature of at least 58.3°C (137°F)
(2) attention to proper disposal of hog feces
(3) prohibiting the marketing of garbage-fed hogs
(4) skin testing of hogs with *Trichinella* antigen prior to slaughter

124. Passive immunization is the major means of prevention of which of the following diseases?

(1) Influenza
(2) German measles
(3) Mumps
(4) Viral hepatitis type A

125. Cholera and plague are reportable diseases according to the 1969 International Health Regulations. Other reportable diseases include

(1) malaria
(2) paralytic poliomyelitis
(3) yellow fever
(4) smallpox

126. Increased risk of nosocomial infections has been associated with

(1) major surgery
(2) indwelling catheters
(3) cancer chemotherapy
(4) antibiotic therapy

127. Which of the following infections or infectious agents can be spread by the venereal route?

(1) Herpes simplex virus, type 2
(2) *Chlamydia trachomatis*
(3) *Treponema pallidum*
(4) Molluscum contagiosum

128. Clinical entities that have been strongly linked to infection with Epstein-Barr virus include

(1) pharyngitis, with atypical lymphocytosis and adenopathy
(2) B-cell lymphoma in Africa
(3) nasopharyngeal carcinoma in Asia
(4) hepatocellular carcinoma in Asia

129. Correct statements about hepatitis B virus include which of the following?

(1) The incubation period for hepatitis B is longer than that for hepatitis A
(2) Prevention of hepatitis B infection can be accomplished by means of hyperimmune globulin or vaccine
(3) Hepatitis B virus may persist in the blood for years
(4) Specific diagnostic tests are not available for hepatitis B

130. The spectrum of illness associated with the primary infection caused by herpes simplex includes

(1) encephalitis
(2) keratoconjunctivitis
(3) vesicular stomatitis
(4) asymptomatic infection

131. True statements concerning histoplasmosis include which of the following?

(1) Human infection usually occurs by inhalation of spore-laden dust particles
(2) Inapparent infections of humans are common
(3) The reservoir of infection is soil contaminated with the excretions of chickens, starlings, and bats
(4) Person-to-person spread occurs frequently

132. True statements about rhinovirus infections include which of the following?

(1) The multiplicity of specific serotypes makes development of vaccine impractical
(2) Nasal mucus is a major source of viral contamination of fingers and environmental surfaces
(3) Conjunctival and nasal mucosa are effective portals of entry
(4) Airborne transmission of rhinoviruses is a major route of spread

133. True statements concerning a vaccine for AIDS include which of the following?

(1) Recombinant DNA technology is being pursued for development of vaccine
(2) Biologic and genetic stability of the viral antigens is crucial if a vaccine is to succeed
(3) Private sector development of vaccine may be inhibited by uncertainties regarding the market for vaccine and product liability
(4) The most promising route for production of vaccine appears to be through culture of attenuated virus in ovary cells of Chinese hamsters

134. Prevention of human brucellosis depends on

(1) pasteurization of dairy products derived from goats, sheep, or cows
(2) treatment of human cases
(3) surveillance of infection in livestock
(4) immunization of farmers and slaughterhouse workers

135. True statements concerning malaria include that

(1) four species of the infectious agent cause human malaria
(2) chemoprophylaxis is highly effective in preventing symptomatic illness
(3) residual insecticides have been a major control measure
(4) falciparum malaria has a case-fatality rate of 50 percent in untreated children

SUMMARY OF DIRECTIONS

A	B	C	D	E
1,2,3	1,3	2,4	4	All are
only	only	only	only	correct

136. Respiratory syncytial virus is an important nosocomial pathogen on pediatric wards because

(1) surfaces are readily contaminated by virus
(2) viral shedding is prolonged
(3) hospital staff may become infected
(4) infected infants with congenital heart disease have high mortality

137. Giardiasis, which affects children more often than adults, occurs on a worldwide basis and is often associated with

(1) waterborne transmission
(2) asymptomatic carriage
(3) bloating, abdominal cramps, and diarrhea
(4) invasion of colonic mucosa

138. In order for children to enter school, most states in the United States require proof of immunization against which of the following infections?

(1) Measles
(2) Poliomyelitis
(3) Diphtheria
(4) Rubella

139. True statements regarding dengue fever include

(1) the infectious agent is a protozoan
(2) the incidence has been increasing in the Caribbean
(3) transmission is by infective ticks
(4) hemorrhagic fever with shock is an occasional consequence of infection

140. Diseases that are transmitted chiefly from person to person include

(1) California encephalitis
(2) St. Louis encephalitis
(3) lymphocytic choriomeningitis
(4) meningococcal meningitis

141. Often, visual disturbances and sore throat are the first symptoms in cases of botulism. Other characteristics of this form of intoxication are described by which of the following statements?

(1) In the United States, most cases result from inadequate processing of home-canned foods
(2) The incubation period is usually 12 to 36 hours
(3) Toxins produced by *Clostridium botulinum* are destroyed by boiling
(4) Death is most often the result of the effect of the toxin on the myocardium

142. Which of the following organisms can be transmitted from person to person?

(1) *Ascaris lumbricoides*
(2) *Taenia solium*
(3) *Necator americanus*
(4) *Entamoeba histolytica*

143. Influenza vaccine is generally recommended for which of the following groups?

(1) All persons over 65 years of age
(2) School-age children
(3) All persons with severe pulmonary disorders regardless of age
(4) Pregnant women

144. Adverse reactions reported following administration of pertussis vaccine include

(1) arthus reaction
(2) seizures
(3) hyperglycemia
(4) fever

145. Human carriers are sources of transmission in

(1) diphtheria
(2) histoplasmosis
(3) typhoid fever
(4) Q fever

146. Correct statements concerning upper respiratory infections include which of the following?

(1) Summertime outbreaks of illness characterized by fever, pharyngitis, and conjunctivitis have most frequently been associated with paramyxovirus infection
(2) Treatment with penicillin hastens recovery in children with streptococcal pharyngitis
(3) Patients with viral upper respiratory infections are generally most infectious the day before their symptoms begin
(4) The most common identifiable cause of pharyngitis is group A streptococci

147. Specific antimicrobial therapy is an important part of the control of

(1) tuberculosis
(2) syphilis
(3) leprosy
(4) salmonella enterocolitis

148. Viral infections transmitted from animals to humans include

(1) yellow fever
(2) measles
(3) rabies
(4) cytomegalovirus (CMV)

149. Following a nuclear war, survivors would be threatened by both increased frequency and increased lethality of infectious diseases. Which of the following factors would increase the *lethality* of infections?

(1) Lack of antibiotics, hospitals, physicians, and medical supplies
(2) Dramatic increase in the insect population
(3) Immunosuppressive effects of fallout radiation
(4) Destruction of sanitation systems

150. The case-fatality rate of cholera is currently less than 1 percent. Major factors responsible for this low case-fatality rate include

(1) treatment with tetracycline or other antibiotics
(2) mass immunization in endemic regions
(3) oral administration of glucose-electrolyte solution
(4) chlorination of water supplies in endemic regions

SUMMARY OF DIRECTIONS

A	B	C	D	E
1,2,3	1,3	2,4	4	All are
only	only	only	only	correct

151. Correct statements regarding transmission of hepatitis B include that

(1) vertical transmission is a major public health problem in Asia
(2) vertical transmission can be prevented by hepatitis B immune globulin and hepatitis B vaccine
(3) persons working in dialysis units are at particularly high risk of occupational exposure
(4) transmission is primarily via the fecal-oral route in the United States

152. Hospital employees involved in patient care are at increased risk both of acquiring and of transmitting certain infections. Vaccines recommended for such workers include *All??*

(1) BCG vaccine
(2) typhoid vaccine
(3) pneumococcal polysaccharide vaccine
(4) rubella vaccine

153. Patients with the acquired immunodeficiency syndrome are at risk of infection with a variety of opportunistic pathogens. Agents that are common causes of infection in patients with AIDS include

(1) cytomegalovirus
(2) *Pneumocystis carinii*
(3) *Candida albicans*
(4) *Cryptosporidium*

DIRECTIONS: Each group of questions below consists of lettered headings followed by a set of numbered items. For each numbered item select the **one** lettered heading with which it is **most** closely associated. Each lettered heading may be used **once, more than once, or not at all.**

Questions 154–157

Match each of the diseases below with the pattern of occurrence in day care centers.

(A) Infection affects children in day care, day care center staff, and close family members

(B) Infection is generally inapparent in the children, but symptomatic in adult contacts

(C) Infection is mild in children in day care and in adult contacts, but may cause significant disease in the fetus if pregnant women are exposed

(D) Infection does not occur at an increased rate in day care centers

(E) None of the above

154. Hepatitis A   G

155. Cytomegalovirus   C

156. Giardiasis   A

157. Leptospirosis   D

Questions 158–161

For each description below, match the appropriate arthropod parasite.

(A) *Sarcoptes scabiei*
(B) *Pediculus humanus capitis*
(C) *Pediculus humanus corporis*
(D) *Phthirius pubis*
(E) None of the above

158. Vector for epidemic typhus and relapsing fever   C

159. Epidemics in school children; best treated with a 1% permethrin preparation   B

160. Vector for Lyme disease   E

161. Burrows under the skin   A

Questions 162–165

For each condition below, select the most closely associated causative agent.

(A) Rotavirus
(B) Enterotoxigenic *Escherichia coli*
(C) Norwalk agent
(D) *Shigella sonnei*
(E) *Yersinia enterocolitica*

162. Diarrhea, enterocolitis, mesenteric adenitis   E

163. Infantile gastroenteritis; antigenically related to Nebraska calf diarrhea   A

164. Winter vomiting disease, parvovirus-like agent   C

165. Traveler's diarrhea   B

Questions 166–169

All the illnesses below may be transmitted from person to person during the incubation period. Match the correct incubation period to each illness.

(A) 3 to 7 days
(B) 2 to 3 weeks
(C) 2 to 7 weeks
(D) 6 weeks to 6 months
(E) 6 months to several years

166. Acquired immune deficiency syndrome

167. Chickenpox

168. Hepatitis A

169. Hepatitis B

Questions 170–173

Match each infection below with the intermediate host involved in transmission.

(A) Snail
(B) Swine
(C) Fish
(D) Crab
(E) Dog

170. Paragonimiasis

171. Diphyllobothriasis

172. Toxocariasis

173. Cysticercosis

Questions 174–177

Select the reservoir for each of the diseases below.

(A) Cattle
(B) Humans
(C) Rodents
(D) Ticks
(E) None of the above

174. Candidiasis

175. Plague

176. Brucellosis

177. Enterobiasis

Questions 178–181

Match each of the descriptions below with the correct worm.

(A) *Necator americanus* (hookworm)
(B) *Ascaris lumbricoides* (roundworm)
(C) *Strongyloides stercoralis*
(D) *Taenia solium* (pork tapeworm)
(E) *Trichuris trichiura* (whipworm)

178. Infection follows ingestion of embryonated eggs, which mature into larvae in the intestine, then migrate to the lungs to mature further

179. Infection of man by this worm in the larval stage is termed *cysticercosis*

180. Intestinal autoinfection may lead to increasing worm burden and dissemination

181. Acquired when infective larvae penetrate the skin; main symptoms are due to iron deficiency

Questions 182–185

Match each group of diseases with the correct description.

(A) Bacterial infections
(B) Zoonoses
(C) Person-to-person spread
(D) Viral infections
(E) Arthropod-borne infections

182. Rabies, psittacosis, salmonellosis

183. Influenza, yellow fever, chicken-pox

184. Pneumococcal, streptococcal, brucellar infections

185. Measles, shigellosis, scabies

Questions 186–189

For each situation below, choose the approximate risk of transmission of the human immunodeficiency virus (HIV).

(A) 1/2 or more
(B) 1/10
(C) 1/500
(D) 1/10,000
(E) 1/100,000 or less

186. Risk to a woman of a single episode of penile-vaginal intercourse with an infected (HIV-positive) man not using a condom

187. Risk to a woman of 10 episodes of penile-vaginal intercourse with a man not belonging to any high-risk group, whose HIV serostatus is unknown

188. Risk to a hospital worker following a single needle-stick from an HIV-infected patient

189. Risk to a recipient of a unit of blood from an HIV-positive donor

Questions 190–193

For each disease, indicate the material in which the infectious agent is transmitted from the infected host.

(A) Conjunctival exudate
(B) Lesion exudate
(C) Blood
(D) Respiratory secretions
(E) Feces

190. Syphilis

191. Shigellosis

192. Pertussis

193. Trachoma

Questions 194–197

Various terms and parameters are used in epidemiologic studies of infectious diseases. Match each statement below with the most appropriate descriptive term.

(A) Immunogenicity
(B) Pathogenicity
(C) Contagiousness
(D) Virulence
(E) None of the above

194. Neutralizing antibody develops in 95 percent of people after an attack of measles

195. Febrile respiratory tract disease develops in approximately 80 percent of children infected with influenza

196. Death occurs in approximately 20 percent of cases of pneumococcal meningitis

197. Approximately 50 percent of household contacts of a child who has a common cold become infected

Questions 198–201

Choose the most likely infectious agent for each description of the events following consumption of food.

(A) Staphylococcal enterotoxin
(B) *Clostridium botulinum* toxin
(C) Enterotoxic *Escherichia coli*
(D) *Clostridium perfringens*
(E) *Salmonella typhimurium*

198. Within 4 hours after attending a church supper, 25 persons report the abrupt onset of nausea, vomiting, and abdominal cramps

199. One week after arriving in Africa, 16 students develop vomiting, severe diarrhea, and abdominal cramps lasting 2 to 3 days

200. A patient dies of respiratory failure after an illness characterized by weakness, diplopia, and cranial nerve paresis

201. Eight to twelve hours after a school banquet, one-third of the persons who attended develop abdominal cramps and watery diarrhea. These symptoms end within 24 hours

Questions 202–205

For each disease, choose the most effective or principal means of control.

(A) Rat control
(B) Sanitation
(C) Immunization
(D) Vector control
(E) None of the above

202. AIDS

203. St. Louis encephalitis

204. Typhoid fever

205. Tetanus

Communicable Diseases

Answers

96. The answer is C. *(Remington, ed 2. p 2.)* Cytomegalovirus (CMV) is the most common cause of intrauterine infection. The rate of fetal infection with CMV per 1,000 live births is 5 to 25 compared with 0.5 for rubella (except during epidemics), 0.8 to 1 for toxoplasmosis, and 0.1 for syphilis and herpes simplex.

97. The answer is C. *(Last, ed 12. p 297.)* About 6 percent of patients admitted to general hospitals in the United States acquire an infection while in the hospital. University and municipal hospitals generally have higher rates of nosocomial infections than small community hospitals. The incidence is two to three times higher in chronic-disease hospitals compared with acute-care institutions.

98. The answer is D. *(Last, ed 12. pp 190–192.)* HSV-2, the main cause of genital herpes, is currently epidemic in the U.S. Many infections are asymptomatic, which makes it difficult to prevent further spread. Infants acquire the infection from their mothers during vaginal delivery; for mothers with known active HSV-2 infections, caesarian delivery within 4 hours of rupture of membranes in indicated. HSV-2 is not an early sign of AIDS—unlike infections like *Pneumocystis carinii*, its occurrence does not suggest immunosuppression. Neonates with any signs of HSV infection should receive antiviral therapy; one of the goals is to prevent dissemination.

99. The answer is B. *(Benenson, ed 14. p 449.)* An *epidemic* is the occurrence of an illness, in a specific geographic area, that clearly exceeds the normal, expected incidence. *Hyperendemic* indicates a situation in which there is a persistent transmission of a disease among most of a population (as with malaria in certain parts of Africa). *Endemic* indicates the constant presence of a disease in a specific geographic area. *Enzootic* refers to the constant presence of a disease in animals in a specific geographic area. *Pandemic* refers to the worldwide spread of an epidemic disease.

100. The answer is E. *(Benenson, ed 14. pp 69–72.)* The major problems associated with chickenpox are its significant morbidity in children, including its association with Reye syndrome; the reactivation of the virus as herpes zoster in later life; and the high morbidity and mortality in immunosuppressed patients. The case fatality rate of chickenpox in normal children is very low. Malformations from gestational chickenpox exposure are very rare (*rubella* is the disease for which this is the major concern). Infection generally confers lifelong immunity, so reinfection is rare. The *incubation* period during which time the patient is asymptomatic is up to 3 weeks, but the *prodromal* period (of mild symptoms) is short.

101. The answer is B. *(Benenson, ed 14. p 451.)* The incubation period is the duration of time between exposure to an infectious agent and the appearance of the first manifestation of the disease. In contrast, the decubation period is the time from the disappearance of symptoms until recovery and the absence of infectious organisms. The communicable period designates the time when the infected person can transmit the infectious agent to another person.

102. The answer is E. *(Ruldolph, ed 18. p 567.)* For every infant with classic symptoms of cytomegalovirus infection, including microcephaly, chorioretinitis, deafness, hepatosplenomegaly, jaundice, and thrombocytopenia, there are probably 20 infants without symptoms. Neurologic sequelae of intrauterine exposure to CMV include mental retardation, minimal cerebral dysfunction, and sensorineural hearing loss. The prevalence of infection at birth is as high as 2.5 percent in some communities.

103. The answer is C. *(Benenson, ed 14. pp 116–120.)* Diphtheria toxoid, alone or in combination with pertussis vaccine and tetanus toxoid (DTP), induces protective levels of antitoxin that persist for about 10 years. Boosters are required every 10 years after completion of primary immunization in order to maintain protective concentration of antibody. Antitoxin antibodies do not prevent infection of the respiratory tract with *C. diphtheriae* and do not prevent the development of the carrier state. The antibodies are directed against the exotoxin produced by the bacteria, not against the bacteria themselves. Adverse reactions from the toxoid are very infrequent in infants and young children but are more common in adults; therefore, the administration of a reduced dose of toxoid is recommended for children over 6 years of age and adults. The reduced dose is symbolized by a lower case d. It is usually combined with tetanus toxoid as a dT.

104. The answer is D. *(Benenson, ed 14. pp 425–426.)* The infectious agent for epidemic forms of typhus fever is *Rickettsia prowazecki,* which is transmitted from person to person by the human body louse, *Pediculus humanis corporis.* Disruptions of social and economic institutions by war, famine, or natural catastrophes are associated with declining standards of personal hygiene and spread of lice. Even before social and economic recovery after World War II, epidemic typhus was controlled by mass application of DDT powder. This insecticide killed the body lice; thus the transmission cycle was interrupted. Effective antibiotic therapy with chloramphenicol and tetracycline was not available until the early 1950s. *Anopheles* mosquitoes are vectors in the transmission of malaria, not typhus.

105. The answer is B. *(Benenson, ed 14. p 451.)* The secondary attack rate of a disease is the ratio of the number of cases of a specified disease among persons exposed to index cases divided by the total number so exposed. According to the data, 400 cases of pertussis occurred among 4,000 fully immunized children who were exposed to a sibling who had the disease. The secondary attack rate, as a percentage, among fully immunized children after household exposure is therefore

$$\frac{400}{4,000} \times 100\% = 10\%$$

106. The answer is C. *(Greaves, Pediatr Infect Dis 2:284–286, 1983.)* The efficacy of vaccine, or the percentage reduction in the incidence of disease in vaccinated compared with unvaccinated subjects, is given by the expression

$$\text{Protection} = \frac{\text{incidence in unvaccinated} - \text{incidence in vaccinated}}{\text{incidence in unvaccinated}} \times 100$$

$$= \frac{(400/1,000) - (400/4,000)}{400/1,000} \times 100\% = 75\%$$

107. The answer is E. *(Last, ed 12. p 48.)* The relative risk is the ratio of the incidence rates of two groups who differ by some factor—in this instance, immunization status. The relative risk is the ratio

$$\frac{\text{Incidence rate among unimmunized children}}{\text{Incidence rate among fully immunized children}}$$

or

$$\frac{400 \text{ cases}/1,000 \text{ exposed children}}{400 \text{ cases}/4,000 \text{ exposed children}} = \frac{0.4}{0.1} = 4$$

108. The answer is A. *(Benenson, ed 14. pp 450–451.)* The incidence of illness (as a percentage) is the total number of persons who have symptomatic illness divided by the total population at risk, and the calculation is $(312 \div 614) \times 100\% = 50.8\%$.

109. The answer is E. *(Benenson, ed 14. pp 450–451.)* The percentage of cases of German measles that were asymptomatic, or subclinical, is calculated by dividing the number of asymptomatic persons by the total number of infected persons. The calculation is $[207 \div (207 + 312)] \times 100\% = 39.9\%$.

110. The answer is E. *(Benenson, ed 14. pp 450–451.)* Age-specific infection rates were 90 percent in all age groups 0 to 59 years of age, while the rate was 10 percent in persons over 60 years of age. The low attack rate in persons over 60 suggests that this age group had developed immunity to German measles as a result of prior exposure at least 60 years before—since there was uniform susceptibility in persons under 60.

111. The answer is A. *(Benenson, ed 14. pp 234–236.)* The injection of live attenuated measles vaccine induces protective antibodies in 95 percent of susceptible children; this seroconversion, or development of active immunity, persists for over 12 years. Postimmunization encephalitis is very rare (1 per 1 million doses) and subacute sclerosing panencephalitis has not been linked definitely to vaccine use. Leukemia and other conditions associated with immunosuppression are contraindications to the use of live measles vaccine because of the risk of developing severe or fatal giant-cell pneumonia.

112. The answer is C. *(Rudolph, ed 18. pp 485, 1696.)* The most common causes (in decreasing order of incidence) of bacterial meningitis in children 3 months to 6 years of age are *Haemophilus influenzae* type b, *Neisseria meningitidis,* and *Streptococcus pneumoniae.* The latter two bacteria cause most cases of meningitis in adults. *Escherichia coli* K1 and group *B Streptococcus* are the most common causes of neonatal meningitis.

113. The answer is C. *(California Department of Health Services, California Morbidity, no. 44, 1986.)* Most patients with antibodies to HIV have the virus in their lymphocytes. Early hopes that only 10 percent of infected persons would get AIDS were overly optimistic: the risk of developing AIDS continues for years, so that the cumulative risk reaches about 30 to 40 percent in 4 years and may continue to rise thereafter. The ELISA test is very sensitive and specific (both about 99 percent), but in low-risk populations, in which the prevalence of true infection may be 0.1 percent or less, the predictive value is low. False positives cannot occur in patients with AIDS because any positive result would be a true positive. False negatives do, however, occur. Antibody-negative patients can probably transmit the disease because development of antibody positivity takes a few months after exposure.

114. The answer is E. *(Last, ed 12. p 301–302.)* Transmission of bacteria from patient to patient most often occurs via the hands of hospital personnel. Airborne transmission, indirect exposure, and common-source exposure do occur but are much less important than direct spread. Indwelling catheters are an important risk factor for nosocomial infection but are not sources of transmission of infections.

115. The answer is D. *(Mandell, pp 388–389.)* According to recent surveys by the United States Centers for Disease Control, about 40 percent of all nosocomial infections involved the urinary tract. Infections of the urinary tract, surgical wounds, and the respiratory tract composed about 80 percent of all nosocomial infections. Over 85 percent of the urinary tract infections were caused by gram-negative, enteric bacteria.

116. The answer is C. *(Rudolph, ed 18. pp 519–521, 547.)* The pertussis vaccine is associated with relatively frequent side effects, probably because it is a concentrated suspension of whole, killed pertussis bacteria, rather than a toxoid. There is no placental transfer of immunity to pertussis, so immunization is begun as soon as the infant is able to mount any kind of response—2 months of age (with diphtheria and tetanus toxoids) is the current recommendation. Immunity is not developed until after the second injection and lasts only a few years. Thus adults, although they do not develop the classic whooping cough picture, are very often susceptible to pertussis. Protection against diphtheria and tetanus is afforded by immunization with toxoids. Patients who have completed their primary immunization series and have had a booster in the last 5 years are not at risk for tetanus and require neither tetanus immune globulin nor additional tetanus toxoid. Those who need additional tetanus toxoid should get a dT to maintain their immunity to diphtheria.

117. The answer is D. *(American Academy of Pediatrics, pp 426–447.)* Asymptomatic children with positive PPD skin tests should have a chest x-ray. If there are no signs of active disease, they should be treated with isoniazid (INH) 10 mg/kg/per day to a maximum of 300 mg per day, for a period of at least 6 months. In low-risk patients, most tests will be negative, and the chance of tuberculosis is so small that many positive tests will be false positives caused by cross-reacting atypical mycobacteria. For these reasons, annual testing of low-risk children is no longer recommended. Adults with tuberculosis are much more likely to be contagious than children. The finding of any person with tuberculosis or a recent skin test conversion mandates investigation of other members of the household.

118. The answer is E. *(Pickering, Pediatr Clin North Am 35:565–567, 1988.)* *Giardia lamblia* infects the upper small intestine; it does not involve the liver. Many infections are asymptomatic. The most common symptoms are diarrhea, bloating, flatulence, and malaise. Fever is rarely seen with *Giardia* infections, and, unlike *Entamoeba histolytica*, *Giardia* does not invade the intestine or cause bloody diarrhea. The incubation period may range from 5 to 25 days; the average is 7 to 10 days.

119. The answer is A (1, 2, 3). *(Benenson, ed 14. pp 412–413.)* Preventive treatment is treatment of *inactive* tuberculosis, that is, tuberculosis without evidence of disease, and has as its objective the reduction of the incidence of active tuberculosis. Preventive treatment with isoniazid, or isonicotinic acid hydrazide (INH), is recommended for children and young adults whose tuberculin tests are positive, for those who have had contact with persons who have recently converted to tuberculin positivity, and for immunosuppressed persons whose tuberculin tests are positive. Because of the risk of INH-associated hepatitis, preventive treatment with INH is no longer routinely recommended for adults over age 35 and is not recommended for prevention of tuberculosis caused by atypical mycobacteria. In a risk-benefit analysis to assess the potential effectiveness of INH, consideration should be given to the high susceptibility to infection of children under 3 years of age, of adolescents, and of young adults.

120. The answer is D (4). *(Benenson, ed 14. pp 221–222.)* Lyme disease is caused by a spirochete, *Borrelia burgdorferi,* transmitted to humans by the bite of infected ticks. The name comes from the town (Old Lyme, Connecticut) from which the first cases were reported. There are endemic foci on the east coast from Massachusetts to Virginia, and in Wisconsin, Minnesota, California, and Oregon. The hallmark of the disease is the characteristic rash, which begins as a red papule (usually at the site of the tick bite) and slowly spreads outward in an advancing annular fashion. This lesion is called erythema chronicum migrans (ECM). Subsequently, joints (either acute or chronic arthritis), CNS (an aseptic meningitis or encephalitis), and heart (atrioventricular arrhythmias or myopericarditis) may be involved. These complications may be diminished by early treatment with tetracycline or penicillin.

121. The answer is A (1, 2, 3). *(Last, ed 12. pp 216–218.)* Type B *Haemophilus influenzae* is by far the most virulent type and accounts for almost all cases of invasive disease. (Remember: B is for bad.) The most important of these diseases are meningitis, epiglottitis, pneumonia, and periorbital or facial cellulitis, and their occurrence is mainly in children. A vaccine made of capsular polysaccharide conjugated with diphtheria toxoid should be given to children at 18 months of age. (This conjugated vaccine should replace the older polysaccharide vaccine, which was less effective in children 18 to 24 months old.) *H. influenzae* is the second most common cause of acute otitis media in children (after pneumococcus), but most cases are due to nontypable strains, rather than to type B. Because ampicillin resistance is increasingly common, life-threatening *H. influenzae* infections should be initially treated with both ampicillin and chloramphenicol, or with one of the newer cephalosporins, such as cefuroxime, cefotaxime, or ceftriaxone.

122. The answer is D (4). *(Benenson, ed 14. pp 158–162.)* Both tetracycline 500 mg q.i.d. for a week and ampicillin 3.5 g plus probenecid 1 g taken at one time are effective in eradicating non–penicillinase-producing *Neisseria gonorrhoeae.* The single dose therapy has the advantages of improved compliance and infrequent side effects. However, because up to 45 percent of patients with gonorrhea have coexisting chlamydial infection, tetracycline should be considered, in spite of its less convenient dosage schedule and tendency to cause mild gastrointestinal discomfort. (These problems are less severe with doxycycline, but doxycycline is considerably more expensive.) In addition, many authorities recommend combining the treatments, to get the benefits of both. Pregnancy is a contraindication to treatment with tetracycline because of possible effects on the developing teeth.

123. The answer is B (1, 3). *(Last, ed 12. p 412.)* Infection of hogs with nematodes of the genus *Trichinella* can be prevented by ensuring that all garbage and offal fed to the hogs are heat-treated to destroy the cysts or, preferably, by using feed devoid of animal meat, such as grain. Prohibition of marketing of garbage-fed hogs is easier to enforce than inspection to ensure that all garbage is properly cooked. Thorough cooking of pork and pork products so that all the meat reaches at least 58.3°C destroys the encysted larvae. Freezing pork also destroys the larvae if adequate time-temperature schedules are followed. The disease is transmitted by ingestion of larvae in skeletal muscle, not by hog feces.

124. The answer is D (4). *(Benenson, ed 14. pp 71, 169.)* Viral hepatitis type A infection can be prevented by the administration of immune serum globulin. German measles, mumps, and influenza are best prevented by active immunization with vaccines.

125. The answer is E (all). *(Benenson, ed 14. p xxiii.)* The selection of infectious diseases to be reported is usually a matter of local discretion. The reporting of cholera, plague, smallpox, yellow fever, paralytic poliomyelitis, and malaria (as well as viral influenza, louse-borne typhus fever, and louse-borne relapsing fever) is universally required in all countries subject to the 1969 International Health Regulations of the 22nd World Health Assembly. Because of their potential for causing epidemics, cases of these diseases should be immediately reported to local health authorities.

126. The answer is E (all). *(Last, ed 12. pp 298–301.)* Nosocomial (hospital-associated) infections are most frequently due to gram-negative enteric bacteria and *Staphylococcus aureus*. The risk of such infections is greatest in patients who have underlying chronic disease and is increased by invasive procedures that bypass host defenses (e.g., use of indwelling urinary catheters and surgery), therapy that alters the viability of normal flora (use of antibiotics), or therapy that depresses host defenses (cancer chemotherapy, major surgery).

127. The answer is E (all). *(Benenson, ed 14. pp 73, 182, 252, 377.)* Sexual intercourse and other sexual activities have been implicated in the transmission of herpes simplex virus, type 2; *Chlamydia trachomatis; Treponema pallidum;* and molluscum contagiosum. Genital infection with herpes simplex virus, type 2, is of significance because of the risk of severe congenital or perinatal infection to the fetus and newborn. *Chlamydia trachomatis* is the most common cause of nongonococcal urethritis, an infection that is more common than gonorrhea in some parts of the world. Its public health significance in the U.S. is as a major cause of pelvic inflammatory disease (PID, salpingitis), which leads to tubal damage and subsequent infertility or ectopic pregnancy. *Treponema pallidum* is the name of the spirochete that causes syphilis. Molluscum contagiosum is a self-limited skin disease characterized by shiny, umbilicated papules; it is thought to be caused by one of the pox viruses.

128. The answer is A (1, 2, 3). *(Benenson, ed 14. pp 253–254, 260–265.)* Epstein-Barr virus (EBV) has been strongly linked to Burkitt's lymphoma, a monoclonal tumor of B lymphocytes common in African children, and to nasopharyngeal carcinoma, which is particularly common in young Chinese men. EBV also causes infectious mononucleosis, a syndrome that generally includes pharyngotonsillitis, lymphadenopathy, and atypical lymphocytosis. Hepatocellular carcinoma is related to chronic infection with the hepatitis B virus.

129. The answer is A (1, 2, 3). *(Benenson, ed 14. pp 167–177.)* Hepatitis B virus (HBV) infection has an incubation period of 6 weeks to 6 months, compared with 2 to 6 weeks for infections caused by hepatitis A virus (HAV). Specific diagnosis of HBV infection can be made by the detection of hepatitis B surface antigen (HBsAg) in the blood during the acute stage of the infection or by detecting antibodies to a variety of antigens of HBV in the convalescent stage. HBsAg may persist in the blood for many years: the chronic carrier state develops in 10 percent of HBV infections in adults. Chronic carriage of HBsAg is associated with a significantly increased risk of chronic hepatitis, cirrhosis, and hepatocellular carcinoma. Hepatitis B immune globulin (HBIG), a preparation of immune globulin containing high titers of anti-HBs, is an effective means of preventing infection if administered within 72 hours after exposure to HBV. Vaccines made from either highly purified HBsAg derived from plasma of healthy chronic carriers or from HBsAg produced by genetically engineered bacteria have been shown to be highly effective in preventing HBV infection. Administration of HBIG followed by three doses of vaccine is 90 percent effective in preventing vertical (mother to baby) transmission.

130. The answer is E (all). *(Benenson, ed 14. pp 182–185.)* Herpes simplex as a primary infection in early childhood is usually asymptomatic. Overt disease, usually stomatitis with fever, occurs in about 10 percent of primary infections. Severe encephalitis may occur with a primary infection or with reactivation of latent infection. Keratoconjunctivitis may also occur during a primary infection or during reactivation of latent infection.

131. The answer is A (1, 2, 3). *(Benenson, ed 14. pp 186–188.)* Histoplasmosis is an infection caused by *Histoplasma capsulatum,* a dimorphic fungus that grows as a mold in soil and as a yeast in human and animal hosts. The reservoir is soil containing much organic matter, such as the enriched soil that occurs around chicken houses and starling roosts, and in bat caves. The infection is transmitted by inhalation of spores; inapparent infections are extremely common in endemic areas. The disease is rarely transmitted from person to person.

132. The answer is A (1, 2, 3). *(Last, p 151.)* The highest concentration of rhinovirus particles occurs in nasal secretions. Peak viral shedding occurs at the time of maximum symptoms. Rhinovirus is regularly recovered from the hands of infected persons and can be transmitted by inoculation of nasal or conjunctival mucosa. Hand-autoinoculation is much more effective in transmitting rhinoviruses than are aerosols. There are over 100 serotypes of rhinovirus; moreover, reinfection with the same serotype can occur because the infection may stimulate only low levels of serum and secretory antibody.

133. The answer is A (1, 2, 3). *(Francis, N Engl J Med 313:1586–1590, 1985.)* Development of a vaccine against AIDS depends on identification of stable viral antigens—if the antigens are highly variable, the virus will change and vaccinees will no longer be protective. Ovary cells of Chinese hamsters have been used to produce hepatitis B vaccine, but the most promising path towards a vaccine for AIDS involves using recombinant DNA technology to produce pure viral antigens, rather than attempting to develop attenuated viral strains.

134. The answer is B (1, 3). *(Benenson, ed 14. pp 57–59.)* Prevention of human brucellosis depends on pasteurization of dairy products from cows, goats, and sheep; education of farmers and workers in the livestock industry as to dangers of infected animals; and care in handling products from aborted animals. No vaccine for human use is available. Since person-to-person transmission does not occur, treatment of individual cases will not control spread of brucellosis.

135. The answer is A (1, 2, 3). *(Benenson, ed 14. pp 225–232.)* The four species causing human malaria are *Plasmodium falciparum, P. vivax, P. malariae,* and *P. ovale.* Chemoprophylaxis is highly effective in preventing disease in nonimmune persons entering endemic areas. Residual insecticides sprayed on the interior walls of dwellings so as to kill the mosquito vectors that may contact these poisoned surfaces have been highly effective in control programs except where insecticide resistance has developed. Falciparum malaria has a case-fatality rate of 10 percent in untreated children and nonimmune adults.

136. The answer is E (all). *(Feigin, ed 2. pp 1263–1268.)* During epidemics of respiratory syncytial virus (RSV), about one-third of infants hospitalized 1 week (for other reasons) develop symptoms of RSV infection. Although lower respiratory infections are seen mainly in infants, 70 percent of infected adults have an illness more severe than the common cold. Infected hospital staff may transmit the infection to patients, because high titers of virus are shed until after clinical symptoms improve, usually longer than 1 week. Virus persists on skin and surfaces for up to several hours. Neonates, infants with congenital heart disease, and immunosuppressed patients have more severe disease, with mortality of 20 to 40 percent.

137. The answer is A (1, 2, 3). *(Benenson, ed 14. pp 156–158.)* Giardiasis occurs all over the world, and epidemics resulting from contamination of water supplies by the protozoan *Giardia lamblia* have occurred in Russia and the United States. Giardiasis is usually a noninvasive infection of the small intestine and has a spectrum of illness ranging from asymptomatic carriage to severe chronic diarrhea. Unlike *Entamoeba histolytica*, the cause of amebiasis, *G. lamblia* does not invade the colonic mucosa.

138. The answer is E (all). *(Centers for Disease Control, State Immunization Requirements for School Children [1983].)* All 50 states require proof of immunization against measles, rubella, poliomyelitis, and diphtheria in order for children to attend school, although 6 apply the rule only to new entrants. Immunization against mumps is required in 30 states, against pertussis in 40, and against tetanus in 47 in order to enter school.

139. The answer is C (2, 4). *(Benenson, ed 14. pp 99–101.)* Dengue fever is caused by any of four serotypes of flaviviruses. Dengue is endemic in tropical Asia and in East and West Africa. Epidemics have recently occurred in Jamaica, Puerto Rico, Trinidad, and other Caribbean islands where dengue had formerly been endemic. The virus is transmitted by the bites of *Aëdes aegypti* and other species of mosquitoes that become infected by biting an infectious human or monkey. Severe hemorrhagic fever with shock, clotting defects, and high fatality rates occurs in children in hyperendemic areas. Diversion of funds from mosquito control to the military has resulted in an increase in dengue in Central America.

140. The answer is D (4). *(Benenson, ed 14. pp 26–27, 222–223, 242–246.)* Meningococcal disease is transmitted by direct contact with droplets and discharges from infected cases and, more often, carriers. California encephalitis and St. Louis encephalitis are acute, inflammatory diseases in which the causative virus is mosquito-transmitted; and lymphocytic choriomeningitis is caused by an arenavirus acquired from contact with food or dust contaminated with urine, saliva, and feces of infected mice. Person-to-person transmission does not occur in these last three diseases.

141. The answer is A (1, 2, 3). *(Benenson, ed 14. pp 145–148.)* Botulism is an intoxication by the exotoxin produced by *Clostridium botulinum*, a gram-positive, spore-forming bacterium. The incubation period is usually 12 to 36 hours. In the United States, most cases are associated with ingestion of improperly home-canned vegetables, fish, and fruits, especially foods that are slightly acidic. At inadequate temperatures spores are not destroyed, subsequently germinate, and multiply under anaerobic conditions. The toxin is destroyed by boiling for at least 3 minutes; but higher temperatures are needed to kill the spores. Death is usually the consequence of respiratory paralysis or secondary infection.

142. The answer is C (2, 4). *(Benenson, ed 14. pp 5–9, 44, 188, 381–384.)* Eggs of *Ascaris lumbricoides* (roundworm) and *Necator americanus* (hook worm) are not infective when passed in feces. With proper moisture, temperature, and soil type, *Ascaris* eggs undergo embryonization for at least 14 days; and after being ingested, they hatch and begin larval development in the small intestine of the human host. The extrinsic developmental period (time from deposition of egg to the infective larval stage) for *Necator* eggs is 7 to 10 days, during which time the eggs hatch and develop to the infective, larval stage. Humans become infected when these *Necator* larvae enter the lymphatic or cardiovascular systems by penetrating the skin. *T. solium* is the pork tapeworm. Adult worms in the human intestine lay eggs, which are directly infectious, either to other people or to the same host. When ingested, the eggs hatch into larvae and migrate throughout the body, causing *cysticercosis*. *Entamoeba histolytica* is an intestinal protozoan. Infectious cysts are passed in the stool; transmission does not require an extrinsic stage of development.

143. The answer is B (1, 3). *(Centers for Disease Control, Morbidity and Mortality Weekly Report 32:333–337, 1983.)* Influenza vaccine is not recommended for routine use in the entire population because current vaccines produce immunity lasting only 1 to 2 years and are only 60 to 70 percent effective. Periodic changes in the viral antigens also contribute to absence of long-term efficacy of vaccines. High-risk groups include all persons over 65 years of age, persons with chronic heart and lung conditions, and persons with other chronic diseases such as diabetes, neuromuscular disorders, and renal failure. Pregnant women have not been shown to be at increased risk of excess morbidity or mortality during recent epidemics. Routine immunization of school children is not recommended with the current vaccines even though school-age children are the major age group involved in the transmission of influenza in the community. If safe, effective vaccines with long-lasting immunity are developed, school children will be the major target group.

144. The answer is C (2, 4). *(Cherry, Pediatrics 81:939–984, 1988.)* Common adverse reactions after pertussis vaccine include fever, irritability, and significant local reactions in approximately half of the recipients. The frequency of these side effects is reduced significantly by administration of 10 to 15 mg/kg of acetaminophen at the time of vaccination, and 4 hours later. High fever (41°C [105.8°F]) occurs in 1 to 2 percent of children. Brief grand mal seizures occur at a rate of approximately 1/1,750 injections. Vasomotor collapse characterized by pallor and lethargy occurs at a similar rate. Hypoglycemia resulting from the stimulation of insulin released by the vaccine has been reported. Prolonged crying occurs in 5 percent of children. The risk of permanent brain damage is estimated from the British Childhood Encephalopathy Study to be approximately 1/310,000.

145. The answer is B (1, 3). *(Benenson, ed 14. pp 116–118, 187, 310–313, 420–424.)* A carrier is an infected host that harbors and can transmit an infectious agent but is asymptomatic and without signs of the disease. Carriers are important sources of transmission of diphtheria and typhoid fever; the asymptomatic carrier state does not occur in histoplasmosis or Q fever.

146. The answer is C (2, 4). *(Rudolph, ed 18. pp 540, 577.)* Outbreaks of fever, pharyngitis, and conjunctivitis have been linked to transmission of adenovirus in swimming pools. Although the effects of penicillin on the course of pharyngitis have been debated for some time, it is now clear that resolution is hastened by penicillin, at least in children. Although rhinoviruses can be transmitted before the onset of symptoms, patients are most infectious when the symptoms are the worst. Numerous viruses, including adenovirus, herpes simplex, influenza, and parainfluenza viruses can cause sore throats, but the most common identifiable pathogen is easily the group A streptococcus, which accounts for about a third of cases.

147. The answer is A (1, 2, 3). *(Benenson, ed 14. pp 213–214, 340, 377–379, 412–414.)* Specific antibiotic therapy is available for tuberculosis, syphilis, and leprosy. Such treatment reduces the potential for transmission by rendering cases noninfectious more rapidly than would occur as the result of development of natural immunity. In contrast to the above infections, antibiotic treatment of enteric salmonella infections is contraindicated because it may prolong the carrier state and lead to resistant strains. Because of the lack of effective treatment, the lack of vaccines against the over 1,500 serotypes of *Salmonella* responsible for salmonellosis, and the enormous animal reservoir of *Salmonella,* control of human disease is very difficult.

148. The answer is B (1, 3). *(Benenson, ed 14. pp 96–99, 233–237, 310–317, 436–438.)* Yellow fever is enzootic among monkeys in the rain forests of South and Central America and Africa. Humans acquire the disease via bites by virus-infected forest mosquitoes. Rabies is acquired from bites by infected animals, primarily skunks and bats in the United States. Measles has no animal reservoir. CMV infections are acquired by direct person-to-person contact, and by vertical transmission during pregnancy, when the infectious agent crosses the placenta to the fetus.

149. The answer is B (1, 3). *(Abrams, N Engl J Med 305:1226–1232, 1981.)* Among many other factors, lack of medical personnel and supplies and decreased host defenses related to radiation-induced immunosuppression would increase the lethality of infectious diseases after a nuclear war. Many other factors, including lack of sanitation, increases in insect vectors, millions of corpses awaiting disposal, crowding in shelters, and disease spread from domestic and wild animals will increase the spread of disease but have much less effect on the lethality of disease.

150. The answer is B (1, 3). *(Benenson, ed 14. pp 75–79.)* Antibiotics and oral-fluid therapy have been the major factors in reducing the case-fatality rate of cholera. Treatment of cholera with tetracycline reduces the volume and duration of diarrhea, thus reducing the need for intravenous administration of fluids. Glucose-electrolyte solutions for oral administration not only have been shown to be well absorbed and capable of maintaining fluid and electrolyte balance but also have reduced the need for intravenous fluid therapy. An effective cholera vaccine has not yet been developed. In any case, vaccination and chlorination would be expected to reduce the incidence, not the case-fatality rate.

151. The answer is A (1, 2, 3). *(Benenson, ed 14. pp 171–177.)* In some areas of Southeast Asia, the prevalence of the hepatitis B carrier state is 20 percent or more. Vertical transmission from asymptomatic infected mothers to their infants is thought to be the major mode of perpetuation of the high endemic carrier rate because hepatitis B acquired in infancy is much more likely to result in chronic infection than when the infection is acquired later. Chronic carriers are important not only as reservoirs for hepatitis, but also because of their very high risk of hepatocellular carcinoma. For this reason it is essential to screen women at high risk for hepatitis B carriage during their pregnancy, so that the infant can be given hepatitis B immune globulin and hepatitis B vaccine, which have been shown to be 90 percent effective at interrupting vertical transmission of the disease. In the United States, the infection is primarily transmitted horizontally, through exposure to blood or blood products via either needles (e.g., in drug addicts, recipients of factor VIII concentrate, hospital workers) or mucous membranes (via sexual contact). Employees of dialysis centers are among those at highest risk. The fecal-oral route is not an important route of transmission of hepatitis B, although it is for hepatitis A.

152. The answer is D (4). *(Centers for Disease Control, Immunization Against Disease [1983], pp 72–73.)* Routine use of BCG for hospital workers is not recommended. Surveillance of personnel for newly acquired tuberculosis infection by means of routine tuberculin skin testing is preferable to BCG. Typhoid vaccination is not recommended because of the very low incidence of typhoid fever in the United States. Administration of pneumococcal vaccine to all hospital employees is not recommended; however, those who are at high risk of pneumococcal disease because of underlying medical conditions should be immunized. All female employees of childbearing age who work with pediatric patients should be vaccinated with rubella vaccine unless they have serologic proof of immunity. All personnel, of both sexes, including physicians, who have direct contact with pregnant women in the hospital or clinics, should have serological testing for susceptibility to rubella performed and should be immunized if susceptible.

153. The answer is E (all). *(Fauci, Ann Intern Med 100:92–106, 1984.)* Fifty to sixty percent of patients with AIDS are infected with CMV, oral candidiasis, or *Pneumocystis carinii,* often in combination. Other common causes of infection include *Mycobacterium avium-intracellulare, Cryptococcus,* and herpes simplex virus. Many patients are also infected with hepatitis B virus. Persistent or recurrent diarrhea commonly occurs in AIDS patients and may be caused by *Cryptosporidium,* an enteric protozoan that also may infect children in day care centers.

154–157. The answers are: 154-B, 155-C, 156-A, 157-D. *(Benenson, ed 14. pp 156, 214–216. Last, ed 12. p 123.)* Hepatitis A virus spreads readily in day care centers, particularly those caring for toddlers in diapers. It usually causes mild or no disease in the children, but may cause significant morbidity in adult contacts.

Cytomegalovirus (CMV) is very common in children in day care centers; in one study more than half of the children excreted CMV over the course of a year, compared with less than 10 percent of children cared for at home. Most infections are asymptomatic, but infection of the fetus can cause microcephaly, mental retardation, deafness, and death.

Giardiasis affects both children and their adult contacts. Symptoms may be absent, mild, or severe and may include diarrhea, bloating, fat malabsorption, and weight loss. Diagnosis is by identification of cysts or trophozoites in the stool (but false negatives are frequent), or by finding trophozoites in duodenal fluid, either by direct aspiration or with a string test.

Leptospirosis is a systemic illness caused by the spirochete *Leptospira interrogans,* acquired by contact of abraded skin or mucous membranes with fresh water contaminated with the urine of infected animals. Transmission from person to person is rare. Doxycycline is effective treatment when given early in the course.

158–161. The answers are: 158-C, 159-B, 160-E, 161-A. *(Benenson, ed 14. pp 221, 278, 341. Brandenburg, Am J Dis Child 140:894–896, 1986.)* Sarcoptes scabiei is the name of the mite that causes scabies. The disease is due to the inflammatory response to the mite, which burrows under the skin and deposits eggs and feces. Treatment is with gamma benzene hexachloride (lindane; Kwell).

Pediculus humanus capitis, the head louse, causes epidemics among school children and institutionalized patients. A preparation of 1% permethrin (a synthetic pyrethrin) is the treatment of choice; lindane is a slightly less effective alternative.

Pediculus humanus corporis, the body louse, is the only louse that is an important vector of disease. It is the vector for epidemic typhus and relapsing fever, as well as for trench fever. It is most closely associated with severe poverty and lack of cleanliness.

Lyme disease is caused by a spirochete, *Borrelia burgdorferi,* transmitted to humans by infected ticks. The incubation period ranges from 3 days to a month after exposure; treatment is with tetracycline (in adults) or penicillin (in children).

162–165. The answers are: 162-E, 163-A, 164-C, 165-B. *(Benenson, ed 14. pp 111, 153, 154, 440. Last, ed 12. p 249.)* A syndrome that includes diarrhea, enterocolitis, severe abdominal pain, and mesenteric lymphadenitis that masquerades as appendicitis is caused by *Yersinia enterocolitica*. The infection is also associated with erythema nodosum and with polyarthritis; the incidence is greater in children than in adults. A variety of wild and domestic animals has been found to be colonized with *Y. enterocolitica*, but the epidemiology of the disease in humans is not fully understood.

Up to 50 percent of hospitalized cases of diarrhea in infants under 2 years of age have been shown to be caused by human rotaviruses, of which there are at least three serotypes. They are antigenically related to Nebraska calf diarrhea virus, the virus of epizootic diarrhea of infant mice, and to many other animal rotaviruses.

Winter vomiting disease, or epidemic viral gastroenteritis, has been associated with a group of parvovirus-like agents that can be identified in the feces of infected persons by electron microscopy. These viruses include the Norwalk agent and the antigenically related Hawaii agent. Humans are the only known reservoir for these agents.

Traveler's diarrhea ("turista") is most often caused by enterotoxigenic *E. coli*. It may be prevented by daily doxycycline or trimethoprim (with or without sulfamethoxazole).

166–169. The answers are: 166-E, 167-B, 168-C, 169-D. *(Benenson, ed 14. pp 4, 70, 169, 173, 451.)* The incubation period is defined as the time interval between initial contact with the organism and the first signs or symptoms of disease. Transmission of diseases from person to person is much more difficult to control when there is a prolonged incubation period, during which the patient may unknowingly transmit the disease to others. This is a major obstacle to control of the AIDS epidemic; patients may transmit the human immunodeficiency virus for many years without ever realizing that they are infected. Both hepatitis A (incubation period 2 to 7 weeks) and hepatitis B (incubation period 6 weeks to 6 months) are most infectious in the period preceding clinical symptoms.

Although the incubation period of chickenpox (2 to 3 weeks) is shorter than that of the illnesses above, chickenpox is much more infectious. Therefore, a child who has been exposed to chickenpox 10 to 14 days before being admitted to the hospital — and thus before development of the characteristic rash — can wreak havoc on a pediatric ward by transmitting the virus to immunosuppressed patients. For this reason, children being admitted to the hospital (especially to tertiary centers) should always be questioned about recent exposure to chickenpox.

170–173. The answers are: 170-D, 171-C, 172-E, 173-B. *(Benenson, ed 14. pp 120–121, 275, 382, 390. Last, ed 12. p 411.)* Paragonimiasis is caused by the lung fluke, *Paragonimus westermani*. It has a complex life cycle in which larval stages undergo development in fresh water crabs and other crustacea. Infection occurs by eating infected raw crabs. The disease, which affects the lungs, causing chronic cough and hemoptysis, occurs primarily in the Far East but has recently been reported in the western hemisphere.

Diphyllobothriasis is the disease caused by the fish tapeworm, *Diphyllobothrium latum*, which uses fresh water fish as its intermediate host. One or two percent of infections are complicated by megaloblastic anemia that is due to interference with vitamin B_{12} absorption, or to competition between the worm and the host for dietary vitamin B_{12}.

Toxocariasis is caused by the dog roundworm, *Toxocara canis*. The disease occurs mainly in children as the result of ingestion of soil contaminated with *Toxocara* eggs. Development of the *Toxocara* is incomplete in humans so that the larval stages migrate through the body—hence the term visceral larva migrans.

Cysticercosis is caused by the pork tapeworm, *Taenia solium*. Intestinal infection occurs by eating pork infested by cysts of *T. solium*. The adult tapeworm resides in the intestinal tract from which gravid proglottids (segments containing eggs) are shed in the feces. If the eggs hatch in the intestinal tract, the larvae can migrate throughout the body, often reaching the brain. Cysticercosis is a common cause of epilepsy in Mexico and other third world countries.

174–177. The answers are: 174-B, 175-C, 176-A, 177-B. *(Benenson, ed 14. pp 58, 60–62, 132, 286.)* The reservoir of *Candida albicans* is the human gastrointestinal tract. Candidal organisms, frequently part of the normal flora in the human body, cause disease only when host defenses are impaired as a result of disease, drug treatment, or altered immune response.

Numerous species of wild rodents are the natural reservoir of plague, in which transmission is through the bites of fleas infected with *Yersinia pestis*. While control of urban plague has been achieved in most of the world, plague still exists in rural areas of the United States, South America, Africa, and the Middle East, and in Central and Southeast Asia. The potential of spread from the wild rodent reservoir to domestic rats, and then to humans, still exists.

Cattle, pigs, sheep, horses, reindeer, and goats are the main reservoirs of brucellosis. A systemic disease in humans, brucellosis may be acquired from raw milk or cheese from infected animals. It is also an occupational disease of farmers, abattoir workers, veterinarians, and others who have contact with animals that may be infected. Important economic losses can be caused by brucellosis in domestic animals.

Enterobiasis is an intestinal infection with the pin worm, *Enterobius vermicularis*. The most common symptom is anal itching, particularly at night. There is no animal reservoir, but infective eggs may survive in household dust for up to 2 weeks; hence careful daily sweeping or vacuuming for a few days after treatment may prevent reinfestation.

178–181. The answers are: 178-B, 179-D, 180-C, 181-A. *(Benenson, ed 14. pp 44–45, 188–189, 374–375, 384–385, 403–404.)* Necator americanus, the American hookworm, enters the skin (usually of the foot) in the larval stage. The larvae are carried via lymphatics and blood to the lungs, where they migrate up the airways to be swallowed. They reach maturity and begin laying eggs in the intestine in 6 to 7 weeks. Autoinfection does not occur because the eggs are not infective for 7 to 10 days. Hookworm disease is primarily due to iron deficiency anemia from chronic gastrointestinal blood loss.

The life cycle of *Ascaris lumbricoides* begins when a person ingests infectious eggs. In the intestine these hatch into larvae, which migrate through the portal circulation to the lungs. After that, the life cycle is similar to that of *Necator americanus:* migration through the alveoli to airways, swallowing, and maturation and laying of eggs in the intestine. *Ascaris* eggs also are not immediately infectious; they require about 2 weeks of incubation. Thus ascariasis is also not directly transmissible from person to person.

The life cycle of *Strongyloides stercoralis* is similar to that of hookworm: larvae enter the skin, travel to the lungs, ascend the trachea, are swallowed, and develop into mature, egg-laying worms in the intestine. However, a crucial difference is that the eggs of *Strongyloides* may develop into infective filariform larvae even before leaving the host, and these larvae may pass through the perianal skin, leading to autoinfection and increasing worm burden. This occurs most often in immunocompromised patients.

Taenia solium, the pork tapeworm, is acquired by ingestion of inadequately cooked pork that is infected with taenia cysticerci (''measly pork''). The cysticerci develop into egg-laying adult tape worms in the intestine. However, unlike those of the beef tapeworm (*Taenia saginata*), eggs of *Taenia solium* are infective to humans. The ingested eggs develop into larvae, which then migrate throughout the soft tissues of the body, including the brain, eye, and heart.

Trichuris trichiura, or whipworm, has a relatively simple life cycle: after embryonated eggs are ingested, they develop into larvae, then adult worms. The worms lay eggs that are not infectious for at least 3 weeks; thus person-to-person transmission and autoinfection do not occur.

182–185. The answers are: 182-B, 183-D, 184-A, 185-C. *(Benenson, ed 14. pp 58, 70, 194, 234, 291, 305, 311, 341, 347, 370, 436.)* Rabies, psittacosis, and salmonellosis are zoonoses, that is, infections transmitted from animals to humans. The reservoirs of rabies include domestic and wild canines, cats, skunks, raccoons, bats, and other biting mammals. Psittacosis is a zoonosis involving birds such as parakeets, parrots, pigeons, turkeys, and other domestic fowl. Salmonella species infect poultry, rodents, dogs, cats, and birds: *S. typhi* is an exception in that no animal hosts are known.

Influenza, yellow fever, and chickenpox are caused by viruses. The diseases differ significantly in their clinical manifestations: influenza is an acute respiratory tract infection; chickenpox is characterized by fever and a typical skin rash; and yellow fever is a severe disseminated viral infection with jaundice.

Pneumococcus, Streptococcus, and *Brucella* are genera of bacteria. Microbes of the first two genera are pathogens responsible for respiratory tract infections in humans. *Brucella* is a cause of widespread zoonoses in cattle, pigs, goats, and sheep, but only occasionally causes human disease.

Measles, shigellosis, and scabies can be transmitted directly from person to person. Measles virus is spread in the respiratory secretions of infected persons; shigellosis is easily caused by ingestion of only a few hundred *Shigella* bacteria and can be spread from person to person by the fecal-oral route; and scabies, a skin infection caused by the mite *Sarcoptes scabiei,* is spread by direct person-to-person contact, often during sexual activity.

186–189. The answers are: 186-C, 187-E, 188-C, 189-A. *(Friedland, N Engl J Med 317:1125–1135, 1987. Hearst, JAMA 259:2428–2432, 1988.)* Although we are in the midst of a monstrous AIDS epidemic, it is important to know that the disease is less infectious than many sexually transmitted diseases. The chance of acquiring the virus depends on the infectivity of the virus and the probability that the contact is infected.

The infectivity from a single episode of penile-vaginal intercourse is very roughly estimated to be about 1/500. (The infectivity is probably higher for anal intercourse and is higher for vaginal intercourse in the presence of genital ulcers.) Condoms are estimated to reduce the risk of transmission by about 90 percent. This reduction is relatively small compared with the effect of selection of a sexual partner. The prevalence of infection in men not belonging to any high-risk group is estimated at roughly 1/10,000, compared with 1/20 to 1/2 in men belonging to a high-risk group. Thus the risk of HIV from a single sexual encounter with a man not at high risk is about $1/500 \times 1/10,000$, or 1/5,000,000. The risk from 10 such encounters is approximately 10 times as high, or 1/500,000, still much less than 1/100,000.

The risk of transmission from infected blood depends largely on the size of the inoculum. Two-thirds of blood recipients from infected donors seroconvert, compared with only 1/100 to 1/1,000 persons exposed by accidental needle-sticks or exposures to mucous membrane.

190–193. The answers are: 190-B, 191-E, 192-D, 193-A. *(Benenson, ed 14. pp 281, 348, 377, 395.)* Infectious agents have developed a variety of means of transmission from one host to the next. Syphilis is spread by direct contact with exudates from early lesions of the skin or mucous membranes, or both of these, usually during sexual activity. Such lesions usually contain large numbers of spirochetes. Infection by indirect contact with contaminated objects rarely occurs because of the lack of viability of the organisms outside the body.

During the diarrheal stage of shigellosis, large numbers of bacteria are excreted. The infectious dose for humans is as low as 100 bacteria; thus the disease is highly contagious, especially among young children who practice poor personal hygiene. Poor sanitation that allows contamination of food or water can cause large-scale outbreaks.

Pertussis, on the other hand, is transmitted in the respiratory secretions of infected persons during talking, coughing, sneezing, or singing. Direct person-to-person spread results from inhaling droplets containing the bacteria. Children are most contagious during the initial (catarrhal) stage during which large numbers of bacteria are present in the profuse nasal secretions. The number of bacteria present in respiratory secretions falls rapidly during the second (paroxysmal) stage of the disease.

Trachoma, a chronic infection of the conjunctiva, is caused by *Chlamydia trachomatis* and is spread by contact with infected discharges from the eye. Direct person-to-person spread is the major means of transmission, although indirect mechanical transmission by flies may also occur. Trachoma is one of the major preventable causes of blindness in the world.

194–197. The answers are: 194-A, 195-B, 196-D, 197-C. *(Mausner, ed 2. pp 268–269.) Immunogenicity* is a term that describes the ability of a microbe or purified antigen to induce specific antibody production in a host as a result of infection or immunization. For example, measles virus is very immunogenic because most persons develop neutralizing antibody, which persists for life following a single infection.

Pathogenicity is the capacity of a microbe to cause symptomatic illness in an infected host. The enormous numbers of nonpathogenic bacteria (up to 10^{10} per gram of colonic contents) present in the human body and the normal flora on the human body's external surfaces do not cause disease.

Virulence refers to the severity of illness produced by a microbe and is measured by the percentage of severe or fatal cases. Virulence may vary depending on the defenses of the host; for example, malnutrition impairs defenses against infection. In malnourished children, measles has a case-fatality rate of up to 10 percent compared with less than 0.1 percent in well-nourished children.

Contagiousness of a microbe refers to the ability of a microbe to spread in a population of exposed susceptible persons. The secondary attack rate, that is, the incidence of a disease in contacts of a case, often is used to assess contagiousness.

198–201. The answers are: 198-A, 199-C, 200-B, 201-D. *(Benenson, ed 14. pp 142–152.)* Staphylococcal food poisoning is caused by a heat-stable enterotoxin produced when staphylococci multiply in food. The incubation period is usually 2 to 4 hours, and the illness is characterized by the sudden onset of severe nausea, vomiting, cramps, prostration, and diarrhea.

Botulism is caused by a toxin produced by *Clostridium botulinum*. The toxin, produced anaerobically in improperly processed foods, is neurotoxic, and the illness is characterized by progressive descending muscle paralysis. Botulism may lead to death from respiratory failure.

Food poisoning caused by *Clostridium perfringens* usually has an incubation period of 10 to 12 hours and is characterized by abrupt onset of abdominal colic followed by diarrhea. Vomiting is unusual, and the disease is usually of short duration. Outbreaks result from contamination of food during preparation and by improper cooking and storage; these circumstances allow bacteria to multiply.

Most cases of traveler's diarrhea are caused by enterotoxin-producing strains of *Escherichia coli.* Although the mechanism of action of *E. coli* enterotoxin is similar to that of cholera enterotoxin, disease due to the former is usually not as severe. Disease due to *E. coli* enterotoxin is most common in regions of the world where adequate sanitation and pure water supplies are absent.

202–205. The answers are: 202-E, 203-D, 204-B, 205-C. *(Benenson, ed 14. pp 28, 348, 385–386, 421–423.)* The principal means of controlling the AIDS epidemic is to effect reductions in high-risk behavior. Both antibody testing (to identify persons capable of transmitting the infection) and education (to inform people of which behaviors are most unsafe) are important components of such efforts. In addition, careful screening of donors, testing of the blood supply, and heat treatment of factor VIII concentrates have reduced transmission of the infection through blood products.

St. Louis encephalitis is caused by a virus in the flavivirus family, one of a group of *ar*thropod-*bo*rne ("arbo") viruses. The disease is transmitted by the bite of an infected mosquito. The viruses are difficult to culture; the diagnosis is generally suspected clinically and confirmed serologically. Control of the arboviral encephalitides requires control of the insect vector; in this instance elimination of breeding grounds for mosquitos, destruction of larvae, screening of sleeping and living quarters, and application of residual insecticides.

Unlike other species of salmonella, *Salmonella typhi,* the cause of typhoid fever, is found only in human beings; there is no animal reservoir. *S. typhi* is excreted in the feces of human carriers. Therefore, control of the disease primarily requires adequate sanitation. Sporadic cases continue to occur in the U.S.; these should be investigated by public health authorities, and the actual or probable source of the infection should be identified.

Immunization with tetanus toxoid is the best means of protection against tetanus. Since the causative organism is a normal inhabitant of the intestine of many animals (including human beings), the need for immunization will persist in spite of the present rarity of the disease. Persons who have sustained dirty wounds should receive tetanus immune globulin (TIG) unless they have an up-to-date status of tetanus vaccination (three past doses of tetanus toxoid, the most recent within the past five years).

Chronic Diseases

DIRECTIONS: Each question below contains five suggested responses. Select the **one best** response to each question.

206. All the following statements about cervical cancer are true EXCEPT

(A) mortality due to cervical cancer has been falling steadily in the U.S.

(B) the Pap test involves sampling cervical cells to look for early signs of the disease

(C) there is an increased incidence of the disease among women with multiple sexual partners

(D) there is no known association between cervical cancer and post-menopausal use of estrogen

(E) there is an increased incidence of the disease among women whose mothers used diethylstilbestrol

207. In the United States, exfoliative cytology is the most utilized test for detection of

(A) skin cancer
(B) breast cancer
(C) stomach cancer
(D) colonic cancer
(E) cervical cancer

208. Which of the following statements about colon cancer in the U.S. is true?

(A) It is two times more common in smokers

(B) It is the second leading cause of cancer death in males

(C) It is a rare cause of cancer death in women

(D) There is an increased incidence of the disease in alcoholics

(E) The death rate from the disease has been decreasing steadily for the past 20 years

209. Which of the following statements about the treatment of hypertension is true?

(A) Treating hypertension has been shown to reduce the incidence of stroke
(B) Treating mild-to-moderate hypertension has been shown to reduce the incidence of coronary heart disease
(C) Most persons with hypertension in the U.S. are not aware that they have high blood pressure
(D) No study has ever demonstrated a benefit from treating hypertension in men
(E) No study has ever demonstrated a benefit from treating hypertension in women

210. Which of the following epidemiologic statements about gastric cancer is true?

(A) The incidence of gastric cancer is higher in Japan than in the U.S.
(B) Annual mortality for gastric cancer has been increasing over the last 40 years in the U.S.
(C) The incidence of gastric cancer is higher in smokers
(D) The incidence in women is twice that in men
(E) The incidence is higher in persons with a history of benign gastric ulcer

211. All the following techniques are considered to be useful in screening for cancer in asymptomatic persons EXCEPT

(A) breast self-examination in a 45-year-old woman
(B) mammography in a 45-year-old woman
(C) mammography in a 55-year-old woman
(D) Pap smear in a 55-year-old female smoker
(E) chest radiography in a 55-year-old male smoker

212. A 40-year-old man with a total cholesterol of 300 mg/dl, a triglyceride of 200 mg/dl, and an HDL cholesterol of 40 mg/dl (after an overnight fast) has an LDL cholesterol of approximately

(A) 260 mg/dl
(B) 220 mg/dl
(C) 160 mg/dl
(D) 140 mg/dl
(E) 60 mg/dl

213. All the following are dietary determinants of plasma lipid levels EXCEPT

(A) alcohol
(B) total calories
(C) cholesterol
(D) saturated fat
(E) vitamin E

214. All the following statements about blindness are true EXCEPT

(A) cataracts cause between one-third and one-half of the cases of blindness in the third world
(B) glaucoma is the most important cause of blindness among blacks in the U.S.
(C) persons with severe myopia are at an increased risk of retinal detachment
(D) proliferative retinopathy is the most common cause of blindness among persons with type I (juvenile-onset, insulin-dependent) diabetes
(E) trachoma is the most common cause of blindness in persons who live in wet tropical environments

215. Premature loss of life can be defined as years of life lost due to a disease before the age of 65 years. The leading cause of premature loss of life in the U.S. is

(A) coronary heart disease
(B) cancer
(C) stroke
(D) congenital heart disease
(E) none of the above

216. Current techniques for estimating the number of cancers caused by low-level radiation are based in part on

(A) data from women who have undergone mammography
(B) data from atomic bomb victims
(C) the Ames model
(D) cohort studies of x-ray technicians
(E) none of the above

217. In the United States, the dominant forms of fatal cancers for men aged 15 to 34 are

(A) bronchogenic and prostatic carcinomas
(B) leukemia and brain tumors
(C) lymphoid and colonic tumors
(D) colonic tumors and melanoma
(E) gastric and colonic tumors

218. Dementia is characterized by

(A) an incidence that peaks in persons aged 60 to 70 years and then declines
(B) an incidence that peaks in persons aged 70 to 80 years and then declines
(C) a prevalence of about 5 percent among persons older than 60 years in the U.S.
(D) a reversible cause in at least 40 percent of cases
(E) none of the above

219. Which of the following statements about microcytic anemia in the U.S. is true?

(A) It usually has a genetic cause in black children
(B) It is rarely caused by a dietary deficiency in men
(C) It is rarely caused by a dietary deficiency in women
(D) It is more common in formula-fed than breast-fed infants
(E) It is not associated with pica

220. The ratio of the prevalence of type I (insulin-dependent) diabetes mellitus to type II (non–insulin-dependent) diabetes mellitus in the U.S. is about

(A) 1:1
(B) 1:4
(C) 1:9
(D) 4:1
(E) 9:1

221. A characteristic demographic feature of rheumatoid arthritis is an incidence ratio of 1:3 that applies to

(A) male:female
(B) blacks:whites
(C) rural:urban inhabitants
(D) high:low socioeconomic status
(E) western:eastern cultures

222. Which of the following statements about valvular heart disease is true?

(A) Coronary artery disease is the most common cause of aortic stenosis in the U.S.
(B) The incidence of rheumatic heart disease in the U.S. has been rising for the past 10 years
(C) Most persons with a history of rheumatic fever are immune to recurrences during group A streptococcal epidemics
(D) Most cases of mitral valve prolapse are asymptomatic
(E) None of the above

223. Asthma is characterized by which of the following?

(A) Age of onset before age 40 years in about 95 percent of cases
(B) Persistently abnormal forced expiratory volume in 1 second (FEV_1)
(C) Greater frequency in girls than boys
(D) Frequent family history of atopy
(E) None of the above

224. Which of the following statements best represents the generally accepted clinical definition of chronic bronchitis?

(A) Three years of cough and at least 2 months of sputum production
(B) Persistent sputum production and cough for at least 2 years
(C) Persistent cough with sputum production for at least 3 months for at least 2 consecutive years
(D) Persistent cough with sputum production for 1 year
(E) Persistent cough for 6 consecutive months for at least 3 years

225. Which of the following statements about emphysema is true?

(A) There is a definitive clinical diagnosis of the disease
(B) Cigarette smokers are twice as likely to develop the disease as nonsmokers
(C) Flow rates on pulmonary function tests resemble those seen in chronic bronchitis
(D) It is equally prevalent in light and heavy smokers
(E) It is associated with the chronic inhalation of coal dust

226. Cystic fibrosis is a genetic disorder of eccrine and exocrine gland function. All the following statements about cystic fibrosis are true EXCEPT

(A) it is the most common genetic disease in whites in the U.S.
(B) it is inherited as an autosomal recessive trait
(C) about 1 in 20 whites are heterozygous for the gene
(D) the diagnosis can be confirmed by demonstrating an absence of chloride in the sweat
(E) about 50 percent of patients survive beyond age 15

227. Which of the following statements about bronchiectasis is true?

(A) It is uncommon in childhood
(B) It is manifested by cough
(C) It is rarely accompanied by fever
(D) It is usually a primary disorder
(E) It is usually a self-limited problem

228. Studies of musculoskeletal disorders in the U.S. have found that all the following statements are true EXCEPT

(A) they are a more common cause of limitation of activity than is cardiovascular disease
(B) back or spine impairments are the most common type
(C) from 60 to 80 percent of the population experiences back pain at some time during their lives
(D) persons who engage in heavy manual work have a greater risk of suffering low back pain than persons who work at sedentary jobs
(E) lower back x-rays and medical examinations are useful ways to screen for workers at high risk of sustaining on-the-job back injuries

229. Major risk factors for coronary artery disease include all the following EXCEPT

(A) an elevated low-density lipoprotein (LDL) level
(B) an elevated high-density lipoprotein (HDL) level
(C) hypertension
(D) cigarette smoking
(E) male sex

230. International studies of cardiovascular disease have shown

(A) that death rates due to coronary artery disease vary by less than 25 percent from country to country
(B) that the death rate due to coronary artery disease is higher in the U.S. than in any European country
(C) that the death rate due to coronary artery disease is similar in the U.S. and Japan
(D) that the death rate due to coronary artery disease has been decreasing more rapidly in the U.S. than in any other country
(E) none of the above

231. Which of the following patients is most likely to have a stroke within a year?

(A) A 70-year-old male smoker with hypertension
(B) A 70-year-old female smoker with hypertension
(C) A 50-year-old woman with mitral valve prolapse
(D) A 50-year-old woman with a recent transient ischemic attack
(E) A 50-year-old man with an asymptomatic carotid bruit

232. Which of the following statements about systemic lupus erythematosus (SLE) is true?

(A) It is more common in whites than blacks
(B) The incidence increases with age
(C) It is approximately ten times more common in women than men
(D) The diagnosis requires a positive antinuclear antibody (ANA) test
(E) It is the most common cause of arthritis in women less than 35 years of age

233. An increased risk of coronary artery disease is most clearly related to elevated levels of which of the following lipoproteins?

(A) Very-low-density lipoproteins (VLDLs)
(B) Low-density lipoproteins (LDLs)
(C) High-density lipoproteins (HDLs)
(D) Triglycerides
(E) Chylomicrons

DIRECTIONS: Each question below contains four suggested responses of which **one or more** is correct. Select

A	if	**1, 2, and 3**	are correct
B	if	**1 and 3**	are correct
C	if	**2 and 4**	are correct
D	if	**4**	is correct
E	if	**1, 2, 3, and 4**	are correct

234. True statements about the incidence of cholelithiasis (gallstones) include that

(1) it is increased in persons with diabetes
(2) it is increased in persons with chronic hemolytic anemia
(3) it is increased in women
(4) it is increased in persons with hypercholesterolemia

235. Compared with persons without kidney disease, patients on chronic dialysis for renal failure have an increased incidence of

(1) infection
(2) suicide
(3) coronary heart disease
(4) hypernephroma

236. The risk of developing cataracts is increased among persons

(1) who have type I (insulin-dependent) diabetes
(2) with a history of alcoholism
(3) who have type II (non–insulin-dependent) diabetes
(4) with an occupational exposure to video display terminals

237. Included among the cancers that have been associated with increasing mortality in the past 25 years are

(1) lung cancer
(2) uterine cancer
(3) pancreatic cancer
(4) stomach cancer

238. Primary hepatocellular carcinoma (hepatoma) is

(1) more common in persons with chronic liver disease
(2) associated with the consumption of raw meat
(3) responsible for 20 to 40 percent of all deaths from cancer in Africa
(4) associated with cigarette smoking

239. Which of the following statements about the relationship between marital status and cancer are true?

(1) The risk of cancer of the cervix is higher in married women compared with single women
(2) The risk of breast cancer is higher in single than in married women
(3) The risk of cancer of the cervix is lower in women who marry late in life than in women who marry earlier
(4) The risk of cancer of the testes is higher in married than in single men

240. A familial aggregation pattern exists for cancer of the

(1) breast
(2) pancreas
(3) colon
(4) larynx

241. Use of postmenopausal estrogens has been consistently associated with

(1) an increased risk of endometrial cancer
(2) an increased risk of breast cancer
(3) a decreased risk of osteoporotic fractures
(4) an increased risk of coronary heart disease

242. Multiple sclerosis (MS) is a chronic demyelinating disease characterized by an increased incidence in

(1) women
(2) persons with certain HLA types
(3) persons who live further from the equator
(4) blood relatives of persons with the disease

243. Cigarette smoking increases the risk of acquiring cancers of the

(1) esophagus
(2) pancreas
(3) larynx and oral cavity
(4) bladder and kidney

244. True statements about blood pressure include

(1) isolated systolic hypertension is defined as a systolic blood pressure above 200 mmHg, with a normal diastolic blood pressure
(2) isolated systolic hypertension is a risk factor for stroke
(3) diastolic blood pressure is a more important predictor of incidence of coronary heart disease than is systolic blood pressure
(4) the prevalence of isolated systolic hypertension increases with age in men and women

245. Worldwide decreases in incidence have been observed in which of the following types of cancer?

(1) Cancer of the cervix
(2) Leukemia
(3) Cancer of the stomach
(4) Cancer of the breast

246. The reasons for the poor 5-year survival rate for pancreatic cancer include

(1) the difficulty of establishing a diagnosis early during pathogenesis
(2) the usual ineffectiveness of radiotherapy
(3) the usual ineffectiveness of chemotherapy
(4) the unsuitability of about 85 percent of patients for resection at the time of diagnosis

247. Statements about the incidence of skin cancer that are true include

(1) it increases with age
(2) it is higher in alcoholics
(3) it is higher in persons who live near the equator
(4) it is higher in women

248. True statements about inflammatory bowel disease include that

(1) the incidence of ulcerative colitis is increased in Jews
(2) total colectomy to prevent malignancy is recommended for all persons who have had ulcerative colitis for more than 20 years
(3) the incidence of Crohn's disease is increased in Jews
(4) total colectomy to prevent malignancy is recommended for all persons who have had Crohn's disease of the colon for more than 20 years

249. Preventable causes of chronic renal failure include

(1) hypertension
(2) recurrent pyelonephritis
(3) interstitial nephritis
(4) polycystic disease

250. Cancers ranking among the top five in children less than 15 years of age in the United States include

(1) cancer of the central nervous system
(2) lymphoma
(3) cancer of the sympathetic nervous system
(4) leukemia

251. Conditions that are associated with an increased risk of pulmonary thromboembolism include

(1) obesity
(2) surgery
(3) use of oral contraceptives
(4) hypertension

252. True statements about myocardial infarction (MI) include that

(1) about 15 percent of MIs are painless
(2) half of the immediate deaths due to an MI occur outside of a hospital
(3) about one in three persons with an MI dies within 1 week
(4) of those who survive an MI, 50 percent die within the next year

253. True statements about osteoarthritis (degenerative joint disease) include that

(1) it is more than twice as common among women as men of the same age
(2) it is about equally frequent in all races among persons of the same age
(3) about 50 percent of persons over age 75 have some degenerative joint disease
(4) hereditary factors are important in Heberden's nodes

254. The prognosis for patients with coronary artery disease is closely related to

(1) dietary intake of cholesterol
(2) left ventricular function
(3) family history of heart disease
(4) degree of coronary artery stenosis

255. The probability that an asymptomatic person will suffer a stroke is increased if the person

(1) has diabetes
(2) is an alcoholic
(3) has electrocardiographic evidence of heart enlargement
(4) has a type A personality

256. In addition to familial aggregation, major epidemiologic characteristics of hypertension include

(1) a lower prevalence among whites than blacks
(2) a higher prevalence among persons with diabetes
(3) a mortality that increases with age
(4) an increased prevalence among persons who consume excessive alcohol

257. Known hazards related to use of oral contraceptives are increased risk of

(1) breast cancer
(2) vaginal cancer
(3) osteoporosis
(4) thromboembolism

258. Though much is still unknown about adult-onset diabetes mellitus, constitutional and environmental factors associated with an increased incidence of the disease include

(1) obesity
(2) age
(3) family history of diabetes
(4) pregnancy

259. Which of the following factors may contribute to development of chronic bronchitis?

(1) Air pollution
(2) Altitude
(3) Occupation
(4) Alcohol abuse

260. Complications of diabetes mellitus include

(1) blindness
(2) pancreatic cancer
(3) limb loss
(4) peptic ulcer disease

261. Inhalation of asbestos particles has been shown to be associated with increased incidence of which of the following disorders?

(1) Pulmonary fibrosis
(2) Peritoneal mesothelioma
(3) Pleural mesothelioma
(4) Emphysema

262. Exposure of nonsmokers to second-hand cigarette smoke may result in

(1) elevation in blood concentration of carbon monoxide
(2) increased incidence of lower respiratory tract infections during the first year of life
(3) eye irritation, headache, nasal congestion, cough
(4) exacerbation of chronic obstructive lung disease

263. True statements about childhood cancer include which of the following?

(1) Mortality has steadily declined in the last 30 years
(2) Acute leukemia accounts for 30 percent of childhood cancer deaths
(3) Survivors of childhood neoplasms are at high risk of developing second cancers
(4) Cancer is the leading cause of death in children 1 to 14 years

264. Prognosis in Hodgkin's disease correlates with factors that include

(1) the stage of disease at the time of diagnosis
(2) the presence of systemic symptoms
(3) the histologic type
(4) the sex of the patient

DIRECTIONS: Each group of questions below consists of lettered headings followed by a set of numbered items. For each numbered item select the **one** lettered heading with which it is **most** closely associated. Each lettered heading may be used **once, more than once, or not at all.**

Questions 265–268

Match each of the descriptions below with the correct type of arthritis.

(A) Gout
(B) Rheumatoid arthritis
(C) Osteoarthritis
(D) Sarcoid arthritis
(E) None of the above

265. Often iatrogenic

266. Usually begins in childhood

267. Most common form of arthritis in the southeastern U.S.

268. One subtype is associated with HLA-B27

Questions 273–276

For each of the age groups below, select the most common cause of death.

(A) Heart disease
(B) Cancer
(C) Stroke
(D) Pneumonia
(E) Automobile accidents

273. 1 to 14 years

274. 15 to 24 years

275. 25 to 44 years

276. 45 to 64 years

Questions 269–272

Match each of the chronic diseases below with the virus with which it has been most closely associated.

(A) Hepatitis A virus (HAV)
(B) Hepatitis B virus (HBV)
(C) Epstein-Barr virus (EBV)
(D) Adenovirus
(E) Cytomegalovirus (CMV)

269. Nasopharyngeal carcinoma

270. Hepatoma

271. Burkitt lymphoma

272. Polyarteritis nodosa

DIRECTIONS: The group of questions below consists of four lettered headings followed by a set of numbered items. For each numbered item select

A	if the item is associated with	**(A) only**
B	if the item is associated with	**(B) only**
C	if the item is associated with	**both** (A) and (B)
D	if the item is associated with	**neither** (A) nor (B)

Each lettered heading may be used **once, more than once, or not at all.**

Questions 277–280

(A) Tobacco

(B) Alcohol

(C) Both

(D) Neither

277. Esophageal cancer

278. Cervical cancer

279. Duodenal ulcer

280. Hip fracture

Chronic Diseases

Answers

206. The answer is E. *(Schottenfeld, pp 893–895.)* Owing to widespread screening with the Pap test, the incidence of cervical cancer has been falling throughout the Western world. Diethylstilbestrol (DES) was used during pregnancy in the 1950s as a way to prevent recurrent miscarriage. It has been associated with an increased incidence of vaginal (clear-cell) carcinoma among daughters.

207. The answer is E. *(Braunwald, ed 11. p 430.)* The efficacy of exfoliative cytology (Pap smear) in permitting identification of asymptomatic precursors to uterine cervical cancer has been demonstrated. Cervical cancer mortality has consistently declined following screening programs based on the Pap smear. Current recommendations are to perform the test every 2 to 3 years following two normal Pap smears in consecutive years.

208. The answer is B. *(Last, ed 12. pp 1133–1158.)* Colon cancer accounts for about 20 percent of all cancer deaths in the U.S. It is the second leading cause of cancer death in men (after lung cancer) and the third leading cause of cancer death in women (after lung and breast cancer). The cause is unknown, but may be related to the action of certain components of the diet, such as saturated fats, on the colonic mucosa.

209. The answer is A. *(Wyngaarden, ed 18. pp 292–293.)* Treating hypertension can reduce the incidence of stroke by up to 90 percent. Most persons with hypertension (70 percent) in the U.S. are aware of their condition. Treatment of hypertension appears to be equally efficacious in men and in women.

210. The answer is A. *(Braunwald, ed 11. pp 1253–1254.)* The incidence of gastric cancer in men is twice that in women. Gastric cancer is common in Japan, Chile, and in parts of Eastern Europe and is much less common in the United States. The steady decline in the incidence of gastric cancer in the United States over the past 40 years has not been adequately explained. Japanese people who have migrated to the United States continue to have a high incidence, but the incidence in their offspring tends more toward the general incidence of the United States. These data are evidence of an environmental etiologic factor in the disease. Also, some evidence has been obtained for a genetic factor: gastric cancer is two or four times more common in relatives of persons who have this disease than in relatives of persons

92

who do not have this disease. Smokers and patients with benign gastric ulcers are not at increased risk.

211. The answer is E. *(Last, ed 12. pp 1151–1155.)* The purpose of a cancer screening technique is to detect the disease at an asymptomatic phase. This is helpful only if early treatment is more effective than later treatment. Detection of lung cancer with radiography in asymptomatic smokers does not meet this requirement.

212. The answer is B. *(Expert Panel, Arch Intern Med 148:37–69, 1988.)* Serum cholesterol is carried on three major types of molecules: low-density lipoproteins (LDLs), high-density lipoproteins (HDLs), and very-low-density lipoproteins (VLDLs). VLDLs are mostly triglycerides; the amount of cholesterol carried on VLDL is approximated as the triglycerides divided by 5. LDL cholesterol is difficult to measure and thus is usually estimated indirectly by the following formula:

LDL cholesterol = Total cholesterol − HDL cholesterol − triglycerides/5

In this example, LDL = 300 − 40 − 200/5 = 220 mg/dl. This is considered to be a very elevated LDL cholesterol (normal is less than 130 mg/dl). Note that the formula is not valid when the triglycerides are greater than about 400 mg/dl.

213. The answer is E. *(Braunwald, ed 11. p 1020.)* Many patients with hyper-cholesterolemia can lower their plasma cholesterol levels by reducing the intake of total calories, saturated fat, cholesterol, and alcohol; however, dietary changes, unless they are severe, do not usually lower plasma cholesterol levels by more than 10 to 20 percent. Interestingly, in low-to-moderate quantities (about two drinks per day) alcohol increases the high-density lipoprotein levels (i.e., has a beneficial effect), whereas at higher doses it increases low-density lipoprotein levels (i.e., has a harmful effect). Vitamin E levels in serum are affected by lipid levels; however, the reverse is not true.

214. The answer is E. *(Last, ed 12. pp 1297–1311.)* Chronic infection of the tarsal conjunctiva with *Chlamydia trachomatis* causes scarring of the eyelids and eventual opacification of the exposed cornea. The poorer the hygiene, the greater the chance for reinfection; thus trachoma is the leading cause of blindness among persons who live in dry environments without access to sufficient water for washing. Cataracts are also a common cause of blindness in the third world, because of inadequate access to surgical facilities. In the U.S., the leading cause of blindness among whites is retinal disease, especially senile macular degeneration; among blacks, glaucoma is the most important (and preventable) cause. Persons with high degrees of myopia (nearsightedness) have elongated eyes, with thin retinas that are susceptible to detachment. Type I (and, to a lesser extent, type II) diabetics are at risk for proliferative retinopathy. In this condition, new blood vessels form on the retina; these vessels are fragile and may cause vitreous hemorrhage and retinal detachment.

215. The answer is E. *(Wyngaarden, ed 18. p 35.)* Because they affect young people disproportionately, accidents are the most important cause of premature loss of life in the U.S. Cancer, which also has a relatively high incidence among the young, is second. Coronary disease, the most important overall cause of death, mainly affects older persons. Congenital heart disease is too rare to be an important cause of premature loss of life. In some communities, AIDS is now the leading cause of premature loss of life.

216. The answer is B. *(Rosenstock, p 183.)* The exact risks from low-level radiation, such as that received from mammography, are unknown and must be estimated from available data on higher levels of exposure. Atomic bomb victims have an increased risk of leukemia, breast cancer, and thyroid cancer. The rates of these diseases have been correlated with approximate radiation dose from the blast. The Ames model is not used to study the effects of radiation; it is used to test the carcinogenicity of chemical substances (those that cause mutations in bacteria may cause malignant transformations in mammalian cells).

217. The answer is B. *(Robbins, ed 3. p 262.)* Leukemia and brain tumors dominate as the fatal forms of cancer in the United States for men aged 15 to 34. Next most common in this age group are Hodgkin's diseases, testicular tumors, and melanoma. Bronchogenic, gastrointestinal, and prostatic carcinomas are rare causes of cancer death in this age group, but are the most important cancers in older men.

218. The answer is C. *(Braunwald, ed 11. p 130.)* The incidence of dementia continues to rise with increasing age; the incidence is about five times higher in persons older than 80 than in those aged 70 to 79. Most surveys in the U.S. and in Western European countries have found a prevalence of dementia of about 5 percent among persons older than 60. Only about 15 percent of dementias are due to potentially reversible causes, such as depression, drug toxicity, and normal pressure hydrocephalus. The most common cause is Alzheimer's disease, which is usually a diagnosis of exclusion.

219. The answer is B. *(Braunwald, ed 11. pp 1495–1496.)* The most common causes of microcytic anemia in the U.S. are iron deficiency, lead poisoning, thalassemia, and the anemia of chronic disease. Iron deficiency on a dietary basis is the most common cause in children and menstruating or pregnant women. However, iron deficiency is rarely seen on a dietary basis in men; finding it mandates a search for a (gastrointestinal) site of blood loss. Pica (a desire to eat unusual substances) can be a cause of microcytic anemia if it involves eating lead paint chips; sometimes pica (e.g., a desire to eat ice) is even seen as a manifestation of iron deficiency. Although the iron in breast milk is highly bioavailable, it is insufficient to keep pace with growth beyond the first 4 to 6 months of life; breast-fed babies thus require an additional iron source (such as fortified cereal) at that time.

220. The answer is C. *(Last, ed 12. pp 1225–1239.)* The prevalence of diabetes increases substantially with age, and most elderly diabetics have type II diabetes. About 2 percent of all Americans have diabetes; of those over age 70 years, the prevalence is about 10 percent. Because type II diabetes can be relatively asymptomatic, up to half of all diabetics may be undiagnosed.

221. The answer is A. *(Braunwald, ed 11. p 1423.)* Rheumatoid arthritis afflicts women three times more than men. Its highest incidence is in the fourth and fifth decades of life. Differences in race, geographical residence, and social, economic, or cultural characteristics have not been related to the prevalence of this systemic disease of unknown cause.

222. The answer is D. *(Braunwald, ed 11. pp 956–970.)* Although rheumatic heart disease is still a major problem in many developing countries, its incidence in the U.S. has been declining for many years. Persons with a history of rheumatic fever are at a substantially increased risk of recurrence, and prophylactic therapy (such as monthly injections of benzathine penicillin) is recommended. Coronary artery disease does not cause any form of valvular heart disease, though it may cause mitral regurgitation with a normal valve because of papillary muscle necrosis. Echocardiographic surveys have found that up to 7 percent of women between the ages of 14 and 30 have mitral valve prolapse; most are asymptomatic.

223. The answer is D. *(Braunwald, ed 11. p 1060.)* Asthma is characterized by reversible bronchospasm. Between episodes FEV_1 may be entirely normal. Its cause is unknown, but may be related to intrinsic (stress) or extrinsic (allergies) factors. Pulmonary infections in infancy, especially bronchiolitis due to respiratory syncytial virus, are a major risk factor. Almost 20 percent of patients have their first attack *after* age 40 years. Although the disease is more frequent in boys than girls, the sex difference disappears in adulthood.

224. The answer is C. *(Braunwald, ed 11. p 1087.)* The widely accepted clinical definition of chronic bronchitis, as proposed by the American Thoracic Society, is persistent cough and sputum production for at least 3 months in at least 2 consecutive years. Chronic bronchitis, common among habitual smokers, may cause atypical metaplasia and dysplasia of the respiratory epithelium and may cause chronic obstructive disease, cor pulmonale, and heart failure. The classic patient with chronic bronchitis is referred to as a "blue bloater" because of hypoxia and edema.

225. The answer is C. *(Braunwald, ed 11. pp 1087–1095.)* The accepted diagnosis of emphysema requires examination of lung tissue. Along with chronic bronchitis, emphysema causes chronic (irreversible) obstructive airways disease; the two diseases cause similar changes in expiratory flow rates. Smokers are at least ten times more likely to develop emphysema than nonsmokers, and heavy smokers are more likely to do so than light smokers. Inhalation of coal dust is associated with pneumoconiosis, a form of restrictive lung disease.

226. The answer is D. *(Last, ed 12. p 1242.)* Cystic fibrosis is the most common genetic disease in whites in the U.S. (sickle cell anemia is the most common genetic disease in blacks). The incidence is about 1 in 2,000 births; about 5 percent of the white population are carriers of the gene (heterozygotes). The diagnosis can be confirmed by finding elevated levels of chloride (>60 mEq/L) in the sweat. Despite suffering from severe obstructive pulmonary disease, as well as other problems like pancreatic insufficiency, about half of the patients with cystic fibrosis survive beyond age 15.

227. The answer is B. *(Braunwald, ed 11. pp 1082–1083.)* Bronchiectasis is quite common in childhood and either may begin as an infection of the bronchi and bronchioles that causes necrosis or may be the consequence of some abnormal physiologic mechanism that causes abnormal dilatation, poor drainage, and secondary infection. Cough, fever, and production of copious amounts of malodorous sputum are characteristic symptoms of bronchiectasis, which can affect persons of any age or sex. Bronchiectasis may persist as a chronic, smoldering, latent infection.

228. The answer is E. *(Last, ed 12. pp 1277–1279.)* Disorders of the musculoskeletal system are the most common cause of limitation of activity in the U.S., affecting about 12 million persons (about 8 million persons are affected by cardiovascular disease, the second leading cause). Back and spine impairments are the most common type, accounting for about half of these cases. Persons who engage in heavy labor, especially if it involves lifting and stooping, are 50 percent more likely to have back pain than are sedentary workers. X-rays and medical examinations are not reliable ways to identify persons at high risk of sustaining a back injury; strength testing seems to be a better method.

229. The answer is B. *(Braunwald, ed 11. p 1019.)* The most important preventable risk factors for coronary artery disease (CAD) are hypercholesterolemia (especially an elevated LDL level), cigarette smoking, and hypertension. An elevated HDL level is associated with a reduced risk of CAD. Of these three risk factors, however, evidence from randomized trials showing a reduction in CAD is available only for treatment of elevated cholesterol levels.

230. The answer is D. *(Last, ed 12. pp 1159–1163.)* The death rate due to coronary artery disease (CAD) varies greatly from country to country, from a low of about 120 per 100,000 men aged 35 to 74 years in Japan, to a high of nearly 900 per 100,000 men in Finland. Several European countries (Finland, Northern Ireland, and Scotland) have higher rates than the U.S. Finland has the highest death rate due to CAD in the world, perhaps related to a high per capita consumption of animal fat.

The low rate of CAD in Japan (one-sixth of that in the U.S.) is thought to be related to diet. The death rate due to CAD has been declining about 2 percent each year since 1968 in the U.S., the most rapid decline in the world.

231. The answer is D. *(Braunwald, ed 11. pp 1930–1941.)* Transient ischemic attacks are a relatively late manifestation of cerebrovascular atherosclerosis. A patient with a transient ischemic attack has about a 6 percent chance of having stroke within 1 year, much higher than that seen in asymptomatic persons who have one or more of the *risk factors* for stroke. These risk factors include the presence of a carotid bruit, age, hypercholesterolemia, smoking, and especially hypertension. Embolic stroke is a rare complication of mitral valve prolapse, but is commonly seen in persons with atrial fibrillation.

232. The answer is C. *(Wyngaarden, ed 18. p 2012.)* Although systemic lupus erythematosus (SLE) is predominantly a disease of young women, it is much less common than rheumatoid arthritis in this age group. The female:male ratio is about 10:1. The black:white ratio is about 3:1 in the U.S. A black woman in the U.S. has about a 1 in 250 chance of developing lupus in her lifetime. Diagnosis is based on fulfilling at least 4 out of 11 criteria (such as the presence of pleurisy or pericarditis), but does not require a positive ANA test.

233. The answer is B. *(Braunwald, ed 11. pp 1019–1021.)* The exact mechanism by which plasma lipoproteins cause atherosclerosis in the coronary (and peripheral) arteries is unknown. Elevated LDL levels have been clearly associated with an increased risk of coronary artery disease (CAD); elevated HDL levels are associated with a reduced risk of CAD. Definitive evidence linking triglyceride levels with CAD is lacking (VLDLs and chylomicrons are composed mainly of triglycerides).

234. The answer is A (1, 2, 3). *(Braunwald, ed 11. p 1360.)* Gallstones are extremely common; about 20 percent of women over the age of 40 have them. Although most gallstones contain cholesterol, elevated levels of plasma cholesterol are *not* associated with an increased risk. Not only are diabetics at an increased risk of developing gallstones, they also have an increased morbidity and mortality associated with the disease. Chronic hemolytic anemia predisposes to the formation of calcium bilirubinate gallstones, which are more common in the orient. Additional risk factors for gallstones include age, obesity, and chronic biliary infection.

235. The answer is A (1, 2, 3). *(Wyngaarden, ed 18. p 576.)* Chronic renal failure is associated with accelerated atherogenesis; dialysis does not appear to slow this process. Overall mortality for patients on dialysis is approximately 5 percent per year. Depression is common. Infections with *Staphylococcus aureus,* mycobacteria, and hepatitis B have an increased incidence.

236. The answer is B (1, 3). *(Braunwald, ed 11. p 72.)* Age is by far the most important risk factor for developing cataracts. Both types of diabetes are complicated by early cataract formation, possibly owing to the effect of hyperglycemia on the lens proteins. Other causes include trauma, radiation, and several congenital infections, such as rubella. Exposure to video display terminals causes fatigue and eye strain, much like studying for examinations.

237. The answer is B (1, 3). *(Braunwald, ed 11. p 422.)* In the past 25 years, age-adjusted mortality has increased for certain forms of cancer, including cancer of the lung and pancreas, probably because of cigarette smoking. The mortality of uterine cancer has declined by about 60 percent in that time, mainly owing to increased acceptance and utilization of the Pap test. Mortality from stomach cancer has also declined by 60 percent; the reason is unknown.

238. The answer is B (1, 3). *(Braunwald, ed 11. p 1351.)* Hepatoma accounts for only 1 to 2 percent of cancers in the Western world. But in parts of the world where chronic, lifelong carriage of the hepatitis B surface antigen (HBsAg) is common, such as Africa, hepatoma is the most common cause of death from cancer in adult men. In the Western world, the tumor is more commonly seen in persons with cirrhosis.

239. The answer is A (1, 2, 3). *(Last, ed 12. pp 1149–1150.)* The relationship that exists between marital status and cancer of the cervix may be due to the increased sexual activity that usually accompanies marriage and increases exposure to possible carcinogenic agents. This theory is supported by the fact that prostitutes as well as married women have an increased frequency of cancer of the cervix. Endocrine factors may account for the difference in the risk of breast cancer between single and married women; breast cancer is more common among nulliparous women than among women who have borne children.

240. The answer is B (1, 3). *(Braunwald, ed 11. pp 424–425.)* A higher than normal incidence of breast, cervical, colon, and stomach cancers has been demonstrated in relatives of patients with these cancers. There are certain inherited syndromes (such as Gardner syndrome) associated with a markedly increased risk of colon cancer (nearly 100 percent). A woman who has a first degree relative (mother, sister, daughter) with breast cancer has a threefold increased risk of developing the disease.

241. The answer is B (1, 3). *(Wyngaarden, ed 18. pp 1444–1445.)* Postmenopausal estrogens (PME) are commonly prescribed for the relief of menopausal symptoms (such as hot flashes) and for the prevention of postmenopausal osteoporosis. They do appear, however, to increase the incidence of endometrial cancer by about 3 to 5 times. Fortunately, this is a rare disease (incidence of about 1 per 100,000), and nearly all PME-associated endometerial cancers have been early stages (perhaps because of an earlier presentation with estrogen-induced postmenopausal bleeding). Recently, some have advocated adding progestins to PME regimens to decrease the risk of endometrial cancer. However, the progestins may negate the beneficial effects of PME on serum lipids (estrogens raise HDL levels) and thus reduce the benefits of PME on coronary heart disease.

242. The answer is E (all). *(Braunwald, ed 11. p 1996.)* Although the cause of multiple sclerosis is unknown, its epidemiology has been well studied. Women compose about 60 percent of the cases. In general, the incidence of the disease increases with distance from the equator: the disease is twice as frequent in the northern as in the southern U.S. Certain HLA types, such as B7 in whites and DW2 in blacks, are more common among patients with the disease. First degree relatives (siblings, parents) of patients with MS have an eightfold increased risk of developing the disease compared with the general population.

243. The answer is E (all). *(Braunwald, ed 11. p 425.)* Tobacco-related cancers (mainly lung cancer) cause more than 30 percent of all cancer deaths in the U.S. Smoking cigarettes increases the risk of lung cancer at least tenfold. As more women with a long-term smoking history enter with the highest incidence rate for lung cancer, rates of tobacco-related cancer among women are increasing. Pancreatic cancer is at least twice as common in smokers; oral, laryngeal, and esophageal cancers are also increased, particularly among heavy alcohol drinkers.

244. The answer is C (2, 4). *(Wyngaarden, ed 18. pp 292–293.)* Contrary to common belief, systolic hypertension is as strong a risk factor for cardiovascular disease as is diastolic hypertension. Isolated systolic hypertension (ISH) is defined as a systolic pressure greater than 160 mmHg, with a normal diastolic pressure (< 90 mmHg). The prevalence of ISH increases with age.

245. The answer is B (1, 3). *(Last, ed 12. pp 1136–1137.)* The incidence of cancer of the stomach and uterine cervix has been decreasing worldwide. However, the incidence of leukemia and cancers of the lung, breast, uterine corpus, and prostate are increasing. The decrease in the incidence of cervical cancer has been attributed to use of the Pap smear; the decrease in stomach cancer has not been adequately explained.

246. The answer is E (all). *(Braunwald, ed 11. p 1381.)* Of 100 patients who have cancer of the pancreas, only one to two patients can be expected to survive 5 years after diagnosis. Early diagnosis is difficult. Patients may complain of vague abdominal pain or weakness. Tumors of the body and tail of the pancreas are rarely detected before metastases. About 15 to 20 percent of patients who have tumors of the head of the pancreas are surgical candidates for resection. Radiotherapy and chemotherapy do not prolong life.

247.   The answer is B (1, 3). *(Braunwald, ed 11. p 424.)* Exposure to ultraviolet light is generally accepted to be a cause of skin cancer. Both squamous and basal cell tumors can result from chronic exposure. Although skin cancer (not including melanoma) is by far the most common form of cancer, very few patients with skin cancer (about 1 percent) die of the disease.

248.   The answer is B (1, 3). *(Braunwald, ed 11. pp 1277–1290.)* Both types of inflammatory bowel disease are more common in whites than blacks and Asians. Jews have three to six times the incidence of non-Jews. There is no sex preference. The peak incidence of both diseases occurs between the ages of 15 and 35. There is an increased risk of colonic malignancy associated with ulcerative colitis, especially among those with pancolitis, who have a risk of cancer of about 40 percent after 24 years of the disease. However, prophylactic colectomy is no longer routine. Instead, periodic colonoscopy with biopsy of suspicious areas is recommended. Patients with pancolitis associated with Crohn's disease are at a slightly increased risk of colonic malignancy and should also have periodic colonoscopy.

249.   The answer is A (1, 2, 3). *(Braunwald, ed 11. pp 1155, 1205.)* Many, if not most, cases of chronic renal failure could be prevented with careful medical management of hypertension, treatment of chronic urinary tract infections, and avoidance of nephrotoxins. One type of interstitial nephritis, known as analgesic nephropathy, is mainly seen in persons with a history of chronic headaches or back pain, who have been treated for many years with analgesics such as phenacetin. Polycystic disease is inherited (there are both autosomal dominant and recessive types); there is no treatment.

250.   The answer is E (all). *(Page, ed 3. pp 79–83.)* Cancer is the second most common cause of death in children 1 to 14 years of age in the United States. Leukemia is the most common cause of cancer death in children, accounting for about 30 percent of such deaths. Other common malignancies include tumors of the central nervous system, lymphomas, tumors of the sympathetic nervous system (neuroblastoma), and soft tissue tumors.

251.   The answer is A (1, 2, 3). *(Braunwald, ed 11. p 1105.)* Conditions and periods associated with a high risk of thromboembolism include the postoperative period, use of oral contraceptives, congestive heart failure, the postpartum period, chronic pulmonary disease, fractures or other injuries of lower extremities, obesity, deep venous insufficiency in the legs, prolonged bed rest, and carcinoma.

252.   The answer is A (1, 2, 3). *(Braunwald, ed 11. p 982.)* Approximately 1.5 million persons die of myocardial infarction (MI) or its complications each year in the U.S. Mortality with acute infarction is approximately 35 percent. Most of these deaths occur within a week of the MI; half before the patient reaches a hospital. Of those who survive an acute MI, more than 80 percent live for more than a year. About one MI in seven is painless; the proportion of painless MIs is even higher among diabetic persons and the elderly.

253. The answer is C (2, 4). *(Braunwald, ed 11. p 1456.)* The prevalence of osteoarthritis is similar by sex, although it is slightly more common in men under the age of 45 years and among women over the age of 55 years. Osteoarthritis is almost universal by age 75. It afflicts all races. Heberden's nodes (swellings of the distal interphalangeal joints) are inherited in an autosomal dominant fashion.

254. The answer is C (2, 4). *(Braunwald, ed 11. p 978.)* Prognosis is related to the type and severity of coronary artery stenosis, and the quality of the function of the left ventricle. Critical stenosis of the left main coronary artery, for example, is associated with a mortality of about 15 percent each year. The severity of myocardial ischemia (as reflected by angina or a markedly positive exercise test) is also predictive. Family history of heart disease and cholesterol intake (to a lesser extent) are risk factors for the incidence of coronary artery disease, but are not predictors of its prognosis.

255. The answer is B (1, 3). *(Braunwald, ed 11. pp 1933–1934.)* The major risk factors for stroke are hypertension, diabetes, electrocardiographic evidence of an enlarged heart, hypercholesterolemia, and cigarette smoking. The risk increases when one of the factors is present and is further increased if more than one factor is present. There is no evidence that alcoholism is related to increased risk of stroke; and type A personality, although possibly associated with an increased risk of myocardial infarction, has not been related to an increased risk of stroke.

256. The answer is E (all). *(Last, ed 12. pp 1195–1214.)* In the United States, blacks have a higher prevalence of hypertension than whites. Almost half of all diabetics have hypertension. Alcohol consumption has also been associated with high blood pressure in several studies.

257. The answer is D (4). *(Braunwald, ed 11. p 1833.)* The only well-established hazard related to use of oral contraceptives is increased risk of thromboembolism. Of the changes that occur with the use of oral contraceptives, most are reversible when the drug is discontinued. There is no association between use of oral contraceptives and breast cancer or osteoporosis. The synthetic estrogen diethylstilbestrol (DES) was identified as a transplacental carcinogen: some daughters of women given the drug during pregnancy to prevent miscarriage subsequently developed adenocarcinoma of the vagina and cervix. However, DES is *not* an oral contraceptive.

258. The answer is E (all). *(Braunwald, ed 11. pp 1778–1782.)* Factors that predispose an adult to diabetes mellitus include increased age, familial inheritance, pregnancy, and obesity, the last being considered the most important factor. About 80 percent of adults who have maturity-onset diabetes are obese. Although the precise mode of inheritance is unknown, the genetic association is clear. A person who is over 40 years of age and who has a parent with diabetes has two to four times the risk of developing the disease. For some unknown reason, the risk is greater if the father rather than the mother has diabetes. Overt diabetes may be precipitated by pregnancy.

259. The answer is B (1, 3). *(Braunwald, ed 11. p 1087.)* Contributing etiologic factors in chronic bronchitis include air pollution, occupation, infection, smoking, and genotype. Chronic bronchitis is more prevalent in urban regions where air is often polluted. Workers exposed to dusts and some gases have a higher incidence of the disease. Not only is cigarette smoking the most common single etiologic factor, it also potentiates every other factor. It impairs ciliary motility, inhibits fixation of alveolar macrophages, leads to hypertrophy of the glands, and probably causes poly-morphonuclear cells to release proteolytic enzymes. Alcohol abuse and altitude are not associated with chronic bronchitis.

260. The answer is B (1, 3). *(Braunwald, ed 11. pp 1791–1793.)* Diabetes is the most common cause of blindness in adults up to age 70 years in the U.S. More than half of all nontraumatic amputations occur in diabetic persons with nonhealing limb ulcers or gangrene. Other complications include renal failure, coronary artery disease, and stroke. The average life expectancy of a type I (insulin-dependent) diabetic is 20 years shorter than that of a person without diabetes.

261. The answer is A (1, 2, 3). *(Braunwald, ed 11. p 1069.)* Almost 10 million workers in the U.S. have been exposed to asbestos fibers. Chronic or long-term inhalation of asbestos causes asbestosis, a form of pulmonary fibrosis. Relationships to bronchogenic cancer and to mesothelioma of the pleura and peritoneum have also been shown.

262. The answer is E (all). *(Braunwald, ed 11. pp 858, 1075.)* Passive, or second-hand, exposure to cigarette smoke may lead to increased levels of carbon monoxide. Children born to parents who smoke cigarettes are more likely to develop bronchio-litis and pneumonia in the first year of life than infants of nonsmoking parents. Other exposed nonsmokers may develop conjunctivitis, headache, nasal congestion, and cough. Exposure to cigarette smoke may exacerbate the symptoms of persons with chronic obstructive pulmonary disease (COPD) and angina pectoris. The incidence of lung cancer appears to be increased in nonsmoking persons married to persons who smoke compared with those married to nonsmokers.

263. The answer is A (1, 2, 3). *(Page, ed 3. pp 32, 48–53, 79–83.)* Cancer is second to accidents among the leading causes of death in children between the ages of 1 and 14 years. New treatment modalities for leukemia, particularly the use of combination chemotherapy and prophylactic CNS therapy, have resulted in a dramatic decline in mortality. Acute leukemia accounts for 30 percent of cancers in children, with CNS tumors and lymphoma the other major types. Patients with childhood cancers have a 0.5 percent risk of developing a new primary cancer each year after radiation treatment.

264. The answer is E (all). *(Wyngaarden, ed 18. pp 1014–1022.)* Prognosis of Hodgkin's disease correlates with the stage of the disease at diagnosis. However, weight loss, fever, and chills are usually regarded as unfavorable prognostic signs and symptoms. Histologic types have been associated with their 5-year survival data: patients with the lymphocyte-predominant type have a better survival than those with the other types. Women have a better prognosis than men; the reason is unknown.

265–268. The answers are: 265-A, 266-E, 267-C, 268-B. *(Braunwald, ed 11. pp 341, 1423, 1445, 1456, 1623.)* Gout is caused by the deposition of urate crystals in a joint. It is almost always associated with hyperuricemia, which is frequently caused by diuretic therapy used in the treatment of hypertension or congestive heart failure. It can also be idiopathic (caused by either overproduction or underexcretion of uric acid), or associated with underlying malignancy or renal disease.

Although rheumatoid arthritis is the most common and severe form of arthritis in children, its *usual* onset is between 35 and 50 years of age. Rheumatoid arthritis is more common in women than men, and among relatives of patients with the disease. The cause of this potentially devastating disease is unknown. Certain types of juvenile rheumatoid arthritis are associated with HLA-B27. Other arthritides associated with HLA-B27 include ankylosing spondylitis, reactive arthritis, and Reiter's syndrome.

Osteoarthritis afflicts the majority of all persons over the age of 75 years and is by far the most common form of arthritis in all regions of the U.S.

Although sarcoid may be slightly more common in the southeastern U.S. than in other regions of the country, it is still a rare disease. In addition, only about one-quarter to one-half of all patients with sarcoid have arthritis.

269–272. The answers are: 269-C, 270-B, 271-C, 272-B. *(Braunwald, ed 11. pp 699–703, 1325–1327, 1351, 1439, 1563.)* The hepatitis B virus, a mostly double-stranded DNA virus, has been associated with both hepatomas and polyarteritis nodosa. Hepatomas are most commonly seen among persons who have been lifelong carriers of hepatitis B surface antigen (HBsAg), usually because they were infected in infancy or early childhood. There may be associated integration of the HBV genome into hepatocytes. Polyarteritis nodosa (PAN) is a systemic vasculitis of small- and medium-sized arteries, classically manifested by fever, abdominal pain, and hematuria. The nature of the relationship between the hepatitis B virus and PAN is not clear; however, approximately 30 percent of patients with PAN are HBsAg positive.

Epstein-Barr virus, a double-stranded DNA virus in the herpes family, is the cause of infectious mononucleosis. High titers of antibody to certain of the viral antigens are seen in the vast majority of patients with anaplastic nasopharyngeal cancer (a relatively common cancer in southeast China), and with Burkitt lymphoma in Africa and New Guinea. Interestingly, there does not seem to be a relationship between Burkitt lymphoma and EBV in the United States.

Hepatitis A virus, adenovirus, and cytomegalovirus are not associated with any particular chronic diseases, though CMV infections are more common among persons who are immunosuppressed.

273–276. The answers are: 273-E, 274-E, 275-B, 276-A. *(Last, ed 12. pp 1125–1132.)* Deaths associated with automobile accidents account for about 20 percent of all deaths in children 1 to 14 years old. In this age group, accidents of all types caused almost 50 percent of all deaths. Cancer is the second leading cause of death. One-third of the deaths in the age group 14 to 24 are due to automobile accidents. Cancer is also the second leading cause of death in this age group. The leading cause of death in the age group 25 to 44 years of age is cancer, only slightly ahead of heart disease. Heart disease is the leading cause of death for adults in the age group 45 to 64 years of age. For these adults, cancer is the second leading cause of death and the death rate for stroke exceeds that for automobile accidents. The only infectious disease listed among the ten leading causes of death is pneumonia, which outranks accidents as a cause of death only in infants less than 1 year of age and in adults over 65 years of age.

277–280. The answers are: 277-C, 278-A, 279-A, 280-C. *(Braunwald, ed 11. pp 1242, 1890. Last, ed 12. pp 1151–1155.)* Alcohol and tobacco both cause esophageal cancer. The risk of the disease is increased in smokers about fivefold and in drinkers about tenfold. Persons who both smoke and drink are also at increased risk of oral cancers.

Carcinogens contained in tobacco smoke have been found in cervical mucus, perhaps explaining the increased risk of cervical cancer in smokers. Cigarette smoking increases the incidence of duodenal ulcers and slows their healing. Studies have shown that failure to quit smoking may prevent ulcer healing even in patients who are otherwise appropriately treated. Alcohol is associated with gastritis and gastric ulcer disease, but not with duodenal ulcer disease.

Osteoporotic hip fractures are more prevalent in thin women who smoke and in alcoholics. The biologic explanation for these epidemiologic findings is uncertain. Other important risk factors include advanced age, female sex, and white race.

Occupational and Environmental Health

DIRECTIONS: Each question below contains five suggested responses. Select the **one best** response to each question.

281. Among the following health care workers, the lowest prevalence of hepatitis B virus markers is found in

(A) dialysis staff
(B) blood bank technicians
(C) staff of custodial institutions for the mentally retarded
(D) surgical housestaff
(E) medical housestaff

282. Exposure to benzene has been associated with all the following hematological diseases EXCEPT

(A) aplastic anemia
(B) non-Hodgkin lymphoma
(C) acute nonlymphocytic leukemia
(D) acute lymphocytic leukemia
(E) chronic myelogenous leukemia

283. Carbon monoxide binds with hemoglobin to form carboxyhemoglobin. All the following statements about carbon monoxide are true EXCEPT

(A) the background level of carboxyhemoglobin in the blood is about 0.4 percent
(B) smoking one pack of cigarettes a day increases the background level about tenfold
(C) the affinity of carbon monoxide for hemoglobin is 200 times that of oxygen
(D) carboxyhemoglobin levels of greater than 25 percent can be fatal
(E) a characteristic sign of carbon monoxide poisoning is acrocyanosis

284. The development of neuropathic symptoms is associated with chronic exposure to all the following substances EXCEPT

(A) mercury
(B) lead
(C) arsenic
(D) sulfur dioxide
(E) nitrous oxide

285. Persons at an increased risk of bladder cancer include workers in all the following industries EXCEPT

(A) manufacture of rubber
(B) dyeing of textiles
(C) manufacture of paint
(D) manufacture of steel
(E) printing

286. Which one of the following diseases is found almost exclusively among persons who have worked with or have been exposed to asbestos?

(A) Bronchogenic carcinoma
(B) Byssinosis
(C) Pleural mesothelioma
(D) Laryngeal carcinoma
(E) Alveolar cell carcinoma

287. Hymenoptera species include bees, wasps, hornets, yellow jackets, and fire ants. True statements about hymenoptera stings include all the following EXCEPT

(A) they cause more deaths in the U.S. than do snake bites
(B) most deaths are due to anaphylactic reactions
(C) most deaths occur in persons without a known Hymenoptera allergy
(D) about 10 to 15 percent of persons in the U.S. are allergic to Hymenoptera venom
(E) desensitization with purified venom is effective

288. Exposure to a total body dose of approximately 500 rads (5 grays) of x-rays or gamma rays is characterized by all the following EXCEPT

(A) skin erythema
(B) gastrointestinal toxicity
(C) bone marrow suppression
(D) seizures
(E) death in more than 50 percent of persons

289. Electrical injury can cause all the following EXCEPT

(A) death
(B) acute renal failure
(C) myoglobinuria
(D) carpal tunnel syndrome
(E) vascular thromboses

290. In the United States, the greatest amount of gaseous and particulate air pollution, when measured by weight, is derived from

(A) the combustion of fuels in engines of motor vehicles
(B) forest fires
(C) the industrial production of chemicals
(D) the incineration of solid wastes
(E) mining and smelting processes of the metallurgical industry

291. All the following chemicals have been associated with kidney disease EXCEPT

(A) β-naphthylamine
(B) cadmium
(C) ethylene glycol
(D) halogenated hydrocarbons
(E) lead

292. The substance that causes allergic disease in the most people in the eastern U.S. is

(A) spores of fungi
(B) house dust
(C) venom of insects
(D) pollen from ragweed
(E) animal dander

293. The major environmental source of lead absorbed in the human bloodstream is

(A) air
(B) water
(C) lead-based paint
(D) food
(E) none of the above

294. Symptoms of chronic lead poisoning include all the following EXCEPT

(A) anemia
(B) abdominal pain
(C) wrist drop
(D) hepatitis
(E) renal insufficiency

295. Which one of the following is the major cause of skin cancer due to occupational exposure?

(A) Anthracene
(B) Coal tar
(C) Creosote oil
(D) Radium and roentgen rays
(E) Ultraviolet light

296. Which of the following substances is causally associated with pneumoconiosis?

(A) Sulfur oxides
(B) Nitrogen oxides
(C) Oil fumes
(D) Dust particles
(E) Cigarette smoke

297. Persons chronically exposed to mercury vapor may develop a syndrome called erethism, characterized by

(A) memory loss, insomnia, and personality change
(B) anemia, hypertension, and renal insufficiency
(C) erythrocytosis, hypercoagulability, and stroke
(D) hepatitis, malabsorption, and hypocalcemia
(E) none of the above

298. Which of the following statements about snakebites in the U.S. is correct?

(A) Most deaths are due to rattlesnake bites
(B) Immediate incision and suction of the wound is recommended if the bite occurred within 1 hour
(C) The bitten extremity should be packed in ice
(D) A constricting tourniquet sufficient to obstruct venous return should be applied to the bitten extremity
(E) None of the above

299. All the following statements related to the disposal of toxic chemical waste are true EXCEPT

(A) less than 20 percent of all hazardous waste is disposed of properly
(B) the most common solution to the problem of toxic waste disposal is burning
(C) groundwater is at particular risk
(D) American industry generates more than 200 million tons of hazardous waste per year
(E) of the more than 10,000 landfill sites in the U.S., about half are licensed to handle toxic waste

300. The most common asbestos-related tumor in humans is

(A) bronchogenic carcinoma
(B) carcinoma of the colon
(C) pleural mesothelioma
(D) peritoneal mesothelioma
(E) pericardial mesothelioma

301. Hypothermia, defined as a core temperature of less than 35°C (95°F), is associated with all the following EXCEPT

(A) use of phenothiazines
(B) hypothyroidism
(C) hypoglycemia
(D) exposure to lead
(E) alcohol abuse

302. Prolonged exposure to polyvinyl chlorides in production is associated with each of the following EXCEPT

(A) acroosteolysis
(B) Raynaud disease
(C) lung disease
(D) angiosarcoma of the liver
(E) scleroderma

303. All the following statements about nonionizing radiation are true EXCEPT

(A) it includes radiowave and microwave frequencies
(B) its main adverse effects are related to thermal injury
(C) excess exposure has been associated with an increased incidence of neoplasms of the CNS
(D) excess exposure has been associated with an increased incidence of cataracts
(E) excess exposure has been associated with spermatotoxicity

304. The industry that has the highest accidental death rate in the United States is

(A) manufacturing
(B) construction
(C) mining and quarrying
(D) transportation and public utilities
(E) service

305. All the following statements about occupational health in the U.S. are true EXCEPT

(A) there are over 20,000 toxic substances in use
(B) occupational diseases are responsible for about 100,000 deaths annually
(C) there are about 400,000 new cases of occupational disease annually
(D) occupational exposures are responsible for about half of all deaths caused by chronic obstructive pulmonary disease
(E) occupational exposures are responsible for about 5 to 10 percent of all cancer deaths

306. Rheumatologic conditions associated with occupational exposures include all the following EXCEPT

(A) Raynaud phenomenon
(B) carpal tunnel syndrome
(C) acroosteolysis
✗ (D) systemic lupus erythematosus (SLE)
(E) gout

DIRECTIONS: Each question below contains four suggested responses of which **one or more** is correct. Select

A	if	**1, 2, and 3**	are correct
B	if	**1 and 3**	are correct
C	if	**2 and 4**	are correct
D	if	**4**	is correct
E	if	**1, 2, 3, and 4**	are correct

307. The development of mesothelioma is a dreaded consequence of exposure to asbestos. Asbestos-related mesothelioma is characterized by

(1) a lifetime incidence of about 10 percent among persons with heavy exposure to asbestos
(2) an increased incidence in smokers
(3) an incidence that depends upon the type of asbestos fiber
(4) a mean latency of about 10 years after exposure

308. The early effects of excess exposure to carbon monoxide include

(1) headache
(2) giddiness
(3) tinnitus
(4) nausea

309. The effects in humans of consumption of water containing fluoride at concentrations that vary between 1.0 and 4.0 parts per million include

(1) nausea, vomiting, diarrhea, and abdominal pain
(2) mottling of the teeth
(3) tetany as a consequence of hypocalcemia
(4) an increased resistance of teeth to decay

310. Which of the following persons are likely to have occupational exposure to asbestos?

(1) Automobile repair workers
(2) Boiler makers
(3) Roofers
(4) Shipyard workers

311. True statements about threshold limit values (TLVs) include

(1) threshold limit values have been established based on industrial experience and on experimental studies on humans and laboratory animals
(2) threshold limit values have been established for a variety of different chemical exposures in the workplace
(3) threshold limit values have been established for heat and noise
(4) the principal applications of threshold limit values are in the determination of the origin of work-related physical disabilities

312. Medical surveillance for workers exposed continuously during each work day to vapors of carbon tetrachloride (tetrachloromethane) should include

(1) evaluation of alcohol intake
(2) liver function tests
(3) kidney function tests
(4) lung function tests

313. True statements about byssinosis include which of the following?

(1) It mainly occurs in persons in the aluminum smelting industry
(2) It affects mainly persons with hyperreactive airways
(3) It classically becomes more symptomatic later in the work week
(4) It causes bronchoconstriction and cough

314. True statements about pneumoconiosis of coal workers include which of the following?

(1) Progressive massive fibrosis occurs in a minority of coal workers who have pneumoconiosis
(2) Inhalation of anthracite (hard coal) dust is more dangerous than inhalation of bituminous (soft coal) dust
(3) Generally, small dust particles cause more scar formation than large dust particles
(4) The causative agent is the silica contained in coal dust

315. An outstanding sign of poisoning by a polychlorinated biphenyl (PCB) compound is a brown discoloration of the fingertips and fingernails. Other signs include

(1) the eruption of acne lesions on the face
(2) swelling of the joints
(3) visual disturbances
(4) ataxia

316. True statements about coal workers' pneumoconiosis (black lung) include which of the following?

(1) Development appears to be independent of duration of exposure to coal dust
(2) Only nonsmokers are covered under the Black Lung Act
(3) It is easy to differentiate from silicosis on chest radiographs
(4) It is usually not associated with functional abnormalities of the lung

317. One type of hypersensitivity pneumonitis is known as farmer's lung, which is characterized by

(1) an immunologic reaction against thermophilic actinomycetes
(2) fever and leukocytosis in its early stages
(3) severe pulmonary fibrosis in its late stages
(4) eosinophilia at all stages

318. Farmers, because of their frequent contact with moist soil, animals, and plants, are likely to become infected by

(1) *Histoplasma capsulatum*
(2) certain serotypes of *Leptospira*
(3) *Aspergillus clavatus*
(4) *Mycobacterium fortuitum*

319. Based on studies of persons who have been poisoned by chronic exposure, methyl mercury has biologic properties that include an ability to

(1) cause atrophy of the cells of the cerebellum and cerebral cortex
(2) accumulate primarily in the liver and kidneys
(3) behave as a mutagenic agent
(4) be eliminated from body tissues mostly by the kidney

320. True statements about frostbite include which of the following?

(1) The affected part should be placed in a water bath at 5°C (41°F)
(2) The affected part should be rewarmed slowly
(3) Rewarming should be stopped if the patient complains of pain
(4) The affected part may be left with a prolonged sensitivity to cold

321. Radiologic findings specific for exposure to asbestos include

(1) bilateral pulmonary fibrosis
(2) unilateral pleural calcification
(3) pleural effusion
(4) diaphragmatic calcification

322. True statements about heat stress include which of the following?

(1) There are four stages: heat fatigue, heat cramps, heat exhaustion, and heat stroke
(2) There is minimal acclimatization to the effects of occupational heat exposure
(3) Heat stroke is characterized by high fever (>41°C [105.8°F]) and delirium
(4) Heat cramps are characterized by episodes of intestinal colic

323. True statements concerning the Occupational Safety and Health (OSH) Act of 1970 and its administration include which of the following?

(1) The OSH Act standards do not apply to all work-related deaths
(2) Workers have a right to know the composition of all hazardous substances they encounter
(3) Coincident with the passage of the OSH Act, there has been an increased interest in job-related health and safety by labor unions
(4) One problem is that new hazards require at least 3 years of hearings before they can be regulated

324. Workers associated with occupational exposure to *inorganic* lead include

(1) battery makers
(2) painters
(3) solderers
(4) gasoline station attendants

325. The key factors involved in the prevention of back injuries include

(1) the prevention of the first injury, since subsequent injuries are more likely to occur
(2) the adjustment of an uncomfortable load once it has been lifted
(3) the development of weight-lifting limits adjusted for the age and physical condition of workers
(4) the requirement of preemployment radiographs of the lumbosacral spine

326. Metals that have been associated with an increased incidence of lung cancer in occupationally exposed workers include

(1) nickel
(2) iron
(3) chromium
(4) silver

327. Loss of hearing due to exposure to noise depends upon

(1) the duration of exposure
(2) the intensity of noise
(3) whether the noise is continuous or intermittent
(4) the spectrum (frequency composition) of the noise

328. True statements about occupational asthma include which of the following?

(1) It accounts for about 50 percent of asthma in adults
(2) It usually improves on the weekends
(3) Diagnosis requires skin testing or serology
(4) It affects mainly persons with underlying hyperreactive airways

329. Human body tissues can be damaged by microwave radiation because this form of energy

(1) can easily penetrate body tissues at long wavelengths (frequencies less than 150 MHz)
(2) when absorbed produces an elevation in temperature that can be damaging to living tissues
(3) causes the surface temperature of the skin to increase at short wavelengths (frequencies over 10,000 MHz)
(4) has ionizing properties that damage cells through formation of free radicals

330. True statements about occupational skin disease include which of the following?

(1) Most cases of contact dermatitis are mediated by an allergic reaction
(2) Allergic contact dermatitis almost always recurs upon reexposure
(3) Chloracne is usually caused by exposure to chlorine gas or hydrochloric acid
(4) A diagnostic feature of chloracne is the presence of yellowish cysts early in the disease

331. A farmworker who presents to an emergency room complaining of excessive salivation and diarrhea should be

(1) questioned carefully about recent foreign travel
(2) questioned carefully about recent chemical exposures
(3) treated with phosphate binders
(4) treated with atropine

332. Health care workers whose fetuses or infants are at special risk include which of the following?

(1) An anesthesiologist who is trying to get pregnant
(2) A pregnant dermatologist who scrubs with povidone-iodine solution
(3) An oncology nurse, in her first trimester of pregnancy, who mixes chemotherapeutic agents
(4) A breastfeeding intensive care unit nurse who wears a lead apron and is exposed to portable radiography

333. Organs seriously affected by carbon monoxide poisoning include the

(1) brain
(2) liver
(3) heart
(4) kidneys

334. True statements about lung diseases caused by inhalation of particles of crystalline silica include which of the following?

(1) They are the most common occupational lung diseases in the world
(2) They can be seen in persons with brief, but intense, exposures to silica dust
(3) Chest radiographs may show eggshell calcifications in hilar lymph nodes
(4) They are mediated by an immunologic reaction

335. The threshold limit value (TLV) is used by industries and government agencies to describe the allowable amount of a toxic chemical to which persons may be occupationally exposed. It is a standard that

(1) has been established for most chemicals in use by industry
(2) is based on average exposure, so that workers can be exposed to levels above the established TLV at times during the work day
(3) takes into account the interaction of a number of toxic chemicals present simultaneously in the same environment
(4) requires a monitoring system to evaluate the levels of the chemical in the worker's environment

336. Ultraviolet (UV) radiation is usually divided into three regions, depending upon the wavelength of the electromagnetic radiation. True statements about UVR include which of the following?

(1) UV-C consists of the shortest wavelengths and is germicidal
(2) UV-B consists of the medium wavelengths and is responsible for sunburn
(3) Both UV-B and UV-C are associated with corneal inflammation and keratoconjunctivitis
(4) UV-A is responsible for suntanning

337. Hospital personnel who provide treatment to patients with iodine 131 may become contaminated by radiation as a result of

(1) accidental contact with urine or fecal specimens of the treated patients
(2) use of a drinking glass used by a treated patient
(3) contact with the bed linens or soiled laundry of the treated patients
(4) breathing the same air as the treated patients

DIRECTIONS: Each group of questions below consists of lettered headings followed by a set of numbered items. For each numbered item select the **one** lettered heading with which it is **most** closely associated. Each lettered heading may be used **once, more than once, or not at all.**

Questions 338–342

Many occupational environments contain airborne substances that cause lung disease. For each disease, select the worker with whom it is associated.

(A) Sugar cane worker
(B) Ceramic worker
(C) Arc welder
(D) Coal worker
(E) Textile worker

338. Berylliosis

339. Bagassosis

340. Byssinosis

341. Rheumatoid pneumoconiosis

342. Siderosis

Questions 343–347

Match each of the workers or hobbyists below with the infectious disease for which they are at risk.

(A) Brucellosis
(B) Hepatitis B
(C) Histoplasmosis
(D) Legionnaires' disease
(E) Sporotrichosis

343. Butchers

344. Gardeners

345. Air-conditioning workers

346. Dentists

347. Spelunkers (cave explorers)

Questions 348–352

Match each of the occupations below with the factor that constitutes the principal hazard to health.

(A) Silica dust
(B) Noise
(C) Vinyl acetate
(D) Hydrogen sulfide
(E) Asbestos

348. Artist

349. Potter

350. Glass manufacturer

351. Sewer worker

352. Foundry worker

Questions 353–357

Certain substances in the occupational environment have been identified recently as carcinogenic agents based on epidemiologic evidence obtained in studies of exposed laboratory animal and human populations. Match each chemical agent with the human target site for cancer.

(A) Skin
(B) Brain, liver
(C) Bladder
(D) Nasal cavities
(E) Hematopoietic system

353. β-Naphthylamine (aminonaphthalene)

354. Benzene (benzol)

355. Nickel

356. Chromium

357. Vinyl chloride

Questions 358–361

Match each of the substances below with the disease or condition most likely to be caused by circumstance of occupational exposure.

(A) Cancer
(B) Chronic bronchitis
(C) Chronic neurologic disease
(D) Pneumoconiosis
(E) Chronic hepatitis

358. Coal

359. Methyl mercury

360. Sulfur dioxide

361. Thallium

Questions 362–364

Match each of the ecological problems below with the associated chemical.

(A) Carbon dioxide
(B) Chlorofluorocarbons
(C) Sulfur oxides
(D) Carbon particulates
(E) None of the above

362. Acid rain

363. Greenhouse effect

364. Depletion of ozone layer

Occupational and Environmental Health

Answers

281. The answer is E. *(Braunwald, ed 11. p 1329.)* Any worker whose job requires frequent contact with blood is at increased risk of exposure to hepatitis B virus. The lifetime risk to such workers is estimated to be between 15 and 30 percent compared with about 5 percent in the general population. Included are dialysis staff, oral surgeons, staff of custodial institutions, and surgeons as well as many nurses in high risk units, blood bank workers, and laboratory technicians.

282. The answer is B. *(Raffle, p 299. Rosenstock, pp 52–57.)* Before exposure to benzene was regulated by federal statute in 1950, it was associated with a dose-dependent incidence of aplastic anemia. Exposure to benzene has also been associated with all the leukemias (with the possible exception of chronic lymphocytic leukemia). There are no clear occupational causes of non-Hodgkin lymphomas.

283. The answer is E. *(Braunwald, ed 11. p 843.)* The smoking of one pack of cigarettes a day will raise the background level of carboxyhemoglobin in the blood from 0.4 percent to about 5 percent. Carboxyhemoglobin blood levels of 4 percent and above generally are regarded as undesirable for humans. In the blood of heavy smokers, the carboxyhemoglobin level ranges from 5 to 9 percent and, at this concentration range, reduces the amount of hemoglobin that can combine with oxygen. Usually, a blood level of 25 percent carboxyhemoglobin produces the major symptoms of anoxia in carbon monoxide poisoning, which, in the absence of therapy, can lead to syncope, coma, respiratory failure, and death. The cardinal (but not omnipresent) sign of carbon monoxide poisoning is a cherry-red color of the lips.

284. The answer is D. *(Braunwald, ed 11. pp 850–855, 1502.)* Exposure to organic mercury can cause an intention tremor, or even delirium (use of mercury in the manufacture of felt hats led to the phrase "mad as a hatter"). Lead poisoning in adults causes peripheral neuropathy and ataxia; in children it can cause irreversible defects in the central nervous system. Long-term exposure to nitrous oxide (usually as a result of abuse) has been reported to cause a neuropathy similar to that seen in pernicious anemia. Exposure to arsenic can cause delirium or even coma. Exposure to sulfur dioxide mainly causes irritation of the mucous membranes.

285. The answer is D. *(Rosenstock, pp 88–89.)* Occupational exposures, especially to aniline dyes and related organic nitrogen compounds, are thought to be responsible for about 20 percent of all cases of bladder cancer (smoking is the other major risk factor). There is usually a long latent period, from 15 to 40 years, between exposure and disease. Workers in the rubber industry are exposed to β-naphthylamine, an antioxidant and a known bladder carcinogen; some physicians recommend that such workers undergo cytologic examination of their urine on a regular basis.

286. The answer is C. *(Braunwald, ed 11. p 1068.)* Mesothelioma, a cancer that develops from the mesothelial cells that cover the pleural and other serous membranes, occurs almost exclusively among persons who because of occupation have been chronically exposed to air containing large numbers of asbestos particles. (Pericardial mesothelioma is not associated with asbestos exposure.) Asbestos particles, each measuring 50 μm in length and 0.5 μm in diameter, generally are regarded as a causative agent for the formation of a granuloma and for the thickening of the parietal and visceral pleurae. Cancer of the bronchus and of the larynx are associated with cigarette smoking. Byssinosis is a pneumoconiosis due to chronic inhalation of textile dusts.

287. The answer is C. *(Braunwald, ed 11. pp 834–835.)* Hymenoptera stings cause about twice as many deaths as do snakebites in the U.S. The venoms contain a variety of allergenic proteins, which can elicit an IgE-mediated anaphylactic response in susceptible victims. Treatment involves local care, and subcutaneous epinephrine if signs of anaphylaxis develop. Since most deaths occur in persons with a known allergy, such persons should carry a kit containing epinephrine and a syringe with them at all times and should use the epinephrine without waiting for symptoms to develop.

288. The answer is D. *(Braunwald, ed 11. p A-6. Raffle, pp 571–575. Rosenstock, p 183.)* Exposure to 400 rads of x-rays (equivalent to 400 millirems of biologic exposure—a rem measures a radiation equivalent in man) is a lethal dose for 50 percent of humans exposed (LD50). Death usually occurs within weeks, secondary to bone marrow failure and infection. Immediate seizures and coma are characteristic of exposure to supralethal doses of radiation (several thousand rads); death is usually rapid. Under the new terminology, 100 rads = 1 gray (Gy), and 100 rem = 1 sievert (Sv).

289. The answer is D. *(Braunwald, ed 11. pp 859–860.)* Body tissues are effective conductors of electricity. Alternating current, which can induce muscular tetany, is especially dangerous. Death can be caused by low-voltage–induced ventricular fibrillation, or high-voltage damage to the central nervous system. Muscle necrosis leading to myoglobinuria can result in acute renal failure. Cataracts can also occur as a late complication. Carpal tunnel syndrome is not associated with electrical injury;

it is caused by entrapment of the median nerve of the wrist, leading to a painful neuropathy that characteristically is most troublesome at night.

290. The answer is A. *(Last, ed 12. pp 576–580.)* The most important cause of air pollution in industrialized countries is combustion of fossil fuels (gasoline, oil) in engines of motor vehicles. Other important sources include industrial processes, heating, and incineration of garbage. Natural phenomena, such as volcanoes and forest fires, may also contribute, especially in less developed countries. Air quality standards have been set for six types of pollutants in the U.S.: total suspended particles, sulfur oxides, carbon monoxide, nitrogen dioxide, photochemical oxidants, and hydrocarbons.

291. The answer is A. *(Rosenstock, pp 80–90.)* Ethylene glycol, found in antifreeze, causes an acute tubular necrosis, usually seen in attempted overdoses. Chronic exposure to cadmium or lead, both of which are used in welding, soldering, and jewelry-making, causes injury to the proximal tubules and may lead to chronic renal failure; acute overexposure has been associated with oliguric renal failure. Halogenated hydrocarbons, such as carbon tetrachloride, cause acute tubular necrosis, especially if exposure is via inhalation. β-Naphthylamine, used in the rubber and dye industries, is associated with bladder cancer.

292. The answer is D. *(Braunwald, ed 11. p 1867.)* Although all the allergens listed are common, the most common is the pollen from ragweed. Ragweed pollen can be found almost everywhere in the eastern United States. Because of its small size (20 to 40 μm in diameter) and light weight, pollen is easily airborne and is widely dispersed by the wind.

293. The answer is A. *(Last, ed 12. pp 598–599.)* Although most lead intake in humans is from ingestion of lead-contaminated food—about 0.3 mg of lead is ingested daily per person—the amount of lead that is absorbed after inhalation of lead-contaminated air is of greater significance because up to 50 percent of inhaled lead, compared with only as much as 10 percent of ingested lead, is absorbed and circulated by the blood. Because modern building codes usually require the replacement of lead domestic water-supply pipes by those made of copper or galvanized iron, drinking water has become a decreasing source of lead poisoning. The intake of lead due to ingestion of lead-based paint is mainly a problem in children.

294. The answer is D. *(Braunwald, ed 11. pp 852–853.)* Lead is one of the most common metals on Earth and has been used throughout the world through much of history. Its use in pigments has led to an epidemic of childhood plumbism (lead poisoning), caused by ingestion of peeling paint or soil containing paint dust. In children, lead poisoning may be entirely asymptomatic, but still severe enough to cause irreversible effects on the developing central nervous system, leading to mental retardation and learning difficulties. There is also an acute encephalopathy associated with lead exposure, which can be treated with chelating agents.

295. The answer is E. *(Braunwald, ed 11. pp 2271–2272.)* More workers are exposed to sunlight than to any of the other carcinogens listed in the question. In occupations related to agriculture, construction, fishing, forestry, gardening, landscaping, road building, and telephone and electric line installation, large numbers of workers are exposed to ultraviolet light. The photosensitizing effects of certain industrial irritants and photosensitizing chemicals such as coal tar or creosols are enhanced by the UV light of the sun so that even a short exposure in the late afternoon is likely to produce severe sunburn.

296. The answer is D. *(Braunwald, ed 11. p 417.)* Pneumoconiosis, a condition in which lung tissue reacts to permanently deposited dust particles, usually occurs as a result of occupational exposure to air containing particulate matter. Anthracosis, silicosis, asbestosis, berylliosis, farmer's lung, and byssinosis are among the more than 30 forms of pneumoconioses that have been described in the literature. Pneumoconiosis usually causes a restrictive lung disease. Sulfur oxides, nitrogen oxides, oil fumes, and cigarette smoke are likely to cause acute bronchospasm or to exacerbate preexisting diseases such as chronic bronchitis and emphysema.

297. The answer is A. *(Braunwald, ed 11. p 853. Raffle, pp 250–256. Rosenstock, p 209.)* Erethism, which may develop after exposure to both organic and inorganic mercury, is characterized by central nervous system (CNS) toxicity. The syndrome usually begins with vague symptoms of fatigue, and anorexia. A dose-related tremor may develop, followed by progressive CNS dysfunction, personality change, and even delirium. Miners, workers involved in the manufacture of disinfectants, fungicides, and wood preservatives, as well as dentists and dental technicians (mercury is found in dental amalgam) are among those exposed. Classically, the disease was seen in mirror makers, who used mercury to coat the backs of the mirrors.

298. The answer is A. *(Braunwald, ed 11. pp 831–833.)* About 800 persons are bitten by poisonous snakes in the U.S. each year; fewer than 20 deaths occur (mainly from rattlesnake bites). Recommended treatment is aimed at preventing lymphatic absorption of the toxin and providing specific antivenin. It includes prompt immobilization and linear incision and suction (if the bite occurred within 5 minutes, and the nearest hospital is more than 30 minutes away). A tourniquet sufficient to obstruct lymphatic return, such as a rubber band, should be used. It is neither necessary nor desirable to obstruct venous return or arterial flow. Ice may worsen tissue damage by cold-induced vasoconstriction and subsequent ischemia.

299. The answer is E. *(Last, ed 12. pp 861–862.)* U.S. industry generates annually over 250 million tons of hazardous waste. Only about 40 million tons of it is being disposed of properly, usually in landfill sites. However, less than 300 landfill sites are currently in use in the U.S. for hazardous waste disposal (of the almost 13,000 landfill sites used for waste).

300. The answer is A. *(Rosenstock, p 42.)* Mesotheliomas of the pleural and peritoneal surfaces are the classic asbestos-related tumors because they are rarely seen in persons never exposed to asbestos. However, it is important to realize that persons with exposure to asbestos are also at a tenfold increased risk of bronchogenic cancer and that this tumor is far more common than mesothelioma. Persons with extensive fibrosis due to asbestosis may have up to a 50 percent risk of developing bronchogenic cancer.

301. The answer is D. *(Wyngaarden, ed 18. pp 2384–2385.)* Hypothermia is a medical emergency that requires prompt rewarming at a rate of about 0.5°C per hour. This can usually be accomplished by passive rewarming (using blankets or sleeping bags). Hypothermia can be caused by a variety of different conditions, ranging from exposure to cold (especially if the subject is also wet) to metabolic abnormalities such as hypothyroidism and hypoglycemia. Phenothiazines interfere with the body's ability to regulate its temperature (and thus can cause either hypothermia or hyperthermia, depending on the ambient temperature); alcohol causes peripheral vasodilation, which increases the rate of heat loss. Exposure to lead is not associated with hypothermia.

302. The answer is C. *(Last, ed 12. pp 631–632.)* Neither polyvinyl chloride (PVC) nor the vinyl chloride monomer from which it is derived have been clearly shown to cause lung disease. PVC exposure causes bone abnormalities (resorption of the distal phalanges with spontaneous fractures) called acroosteolysis. PVC can also cause a nonmalignant form of liver disease with associated portal hypertension.

303. The answer is C. *(Rosenstock, pp 185–186.)* Nonionizing radiation does not cause molecular ionization or disruption of atomic nuclei. It also includes infrared, visible, and ultraviolet light. Heating of susceptible tissues causes the main harmful effects, such as skin burns and cataracts. Spermatogenesis is also adversely affected by the excess temperatures caused by exposure. No increase in neoplasms, with the important exception of dermatologic malignancies, has been documented.

304. The answer is C. *(Last, ed 12. pp 1565–1566.)* Mining and quarrying is the most dangerous industry in the United States. Agriculture is second; about 50 deaths per 100,000 workers occur each year. According to recent estimates, about 109 million disabling injuries and 11,000 deaths occur annually in industrial occupations.

305. The answer is D. *(Rosenstock, pp 1–3.)* Occupational diseases are an important health problem in the U.S. Their diagnosis remains a challenge, partly because the presentations of these diseases are usually not distinguishable from those unrelated to occupational exposures. In addition, there may be a lengthy latent interval between the occupational exposure and the first manifestations of the disease, and clinicians may not ascertain the nature of those exposures. Although certain occupational exposures, such as those to coal and silica dust, are associated with chronic obstructive pulmonary disease, cigarette smoking is responsible for about 90 percent of all deaths due to the disease in the U.S.

306. The answer is D. *(Rosenstock, pp 61–71.)* Occupational exposures have been associated with a wide variety of rheumatologic syndromes. Some, such as Raynaud phenomenon and carpal tunnel syndrome, are thought to be caused by mechanical problems, including vibration and overuse. Others are associated with specific toxicities, such as lead-induced gout and polyvinyl chloride–induced acroosteolysis. The latter condition closely resembles scleroderma.

307. The answer is B (1, 3). *(Raffle, pp 680–683. Rosenstock, p 41.)* The mean latency period from exposure to the development of mesothelioma is 35 years. The disease often develops in the absence of radiographic asbestosis. There are no other known risk factors besides exposure to asbestos. The chrysotile type of asbestos appears to present less risk than other types.

308. The answer is E (all). *(Last, ed 12. pp 683–684.)* The OSHA standard for carbon monoxide exposure is 50 parts per million (ppm), 8-hour time-weighted average based on a healthy population without cardiopulmonary disease. This may be expected to result in a carboxyhemoglobin level of less than 5 percent. Carboxyhemoglobin levels above 10 percent are associated with headache; in the teens, giddiness and tinnitus; and at 20 to 30 percent, nausea and weakness.

309. The answer is C (2, 4). *(Last, ed 12. pp 1478–1484.)* Fluoridated drinking water is regarded as an effective caries-prevention agent only for children during the period of tooth formation, even though mottling (fluorosis) of the teeth occurs in 10 percent of children who consume water containing fluoride at a concentration of 1.0 parts per million (ppm) and in nearly 100 percent of children when the fluoride level is increased to about 6.0 ppm. Drinking water containing 1.0 ppm of fluoride generally is considered safe and a practical public health measure to reduce the incidence of dental caries, and a dietary supplement of fluoride is not needed for prevention of caries unless the drinking water contains less than 0.7 ppm of fluoride. The continuous consumption of water containing large amounts of fluoride can be expected to induce nausea, vomiting, abdominal pain, diarrhea, and tetany because fluoride combines with calcium to form an insoluble complex. This process results in hypocalcemia, which causes tremors, spasms, and convulsions.

310. The answer is E (all). *(Rosenstock, p 242.)* There are many occupations that may involve exposure to asbestos. Asbestos has been used (and is used) extensively in insulation for boilers and pipes, in brakes, and in roofing materials. Construction and demolition workers may also be exposed to asbestos in insulation and flooring. Because exposure to even small amounts of asbestos is a health hazard, such workers should always use respiratory precautions and should not even wear their work clothes home.

311. The answer is A (1, 2, 3). *(Last, ed 12. p 503.)* A threshold limit value (TLV) is based on the time-weighted (for an 8-hour work day) exposure to a substance that is associated with adverse effects. TLVs have also been established for certain physical agents, such as heat; ionizing, ultraviolet, laser, and microwave radiation; and noise by the American Conference of Governmental Industrial Hygienists. While this organization is a private, unofficial agency, it has established TLVs that have been adopted in federal legislative codes. TLVs are determined on the bases of industrial experience and studies in humans and laboratory animals.

312. The answer is A (1, 2, 3). *(Last, ed 12. pp 628–629.)* Damage to the liver and kidneys, nausea, vomiting, anorexia, apathy, mental confusion, and weight loss are among the effects of occupational exposure to the widely used, highly volatile industrial solvent carbon tetrachloride (tetrachloromethane, or CCl_4) at ambient air concentrations of over 100 parts per million (ppm). Entry of CCl_4 as a vapor into the human body can occur readily by inhalation and as a liquid by ingestion, and the absorption of this substance is enhanced when it is ingested concomitantly with fats or alcoholic beverages. Therefore, a prudent medical surveillance program for workers exposed to CCl_4 should include liver and renal function tests and consideration of the alcoholic beverage intake of each exposed worker. In humans, reversible oliguria is a consequence of mild poisoning by CCl_4, whereas in severe cases of poisoning the oliguria progresses to anuria, proteinuria, and hematuria. Since the odor of CCl_4 cannot be detected at low atmospheric concentrations, workers cannot rely on smell to warn them of the presence of hazardous levels.

313. The answer is D (4). *(Raffle, pp 690–705. Rosenstock, p 25.)* Byssinosis, which is derived from the Greek word for *flax*, afflicts persons who work with dusts from certain plants, such as cotton bracts, hemp, and flax. It causes bronchoconstriction, even in persons who do not have hyperreactive airways. It tends to be worst when workers return after a weekend. The first description of the symptom pattern, in 1845, noted, ''All of the workers told us that the dust bothered them much less on the last days of the week than on Monday and Tuesday. The masters find the cause of this increased sensitivity to be in the excesses of Sunday. . . .'' The pathophysiologic explanation for the disease is not known.

314. The answer is A (1, 2, 3). *(Last, ed 12. pp 545–552.)* Usually, pneumoconiosis develops in coal workers who have been exposed for 10 to 20 years to coal dust that varies in size from 0.5 to 5 μm. This condition was noted to occur even in coal workers exposed to dust virtually free of silica. Anthracite dust is more dangerous for two reasons: (1) the smaller particle size causes more extensive scar formation; and (2) anthracite deposits are associated with higher levels of silica dust.

315. The answer is A (1, 2, 3). *(Last, ed 12. pp 663–666.)* The adverse effects of exposure to polychlorinated biphenyls (PCBs) were noted nearly 40 years after industrial utilization of this organic compound. By investigation of mass poisoning by PCBs that occurred in Japan in 1968, ingestion of as little as 0.5 g of tetrachlorobiphenyl was shown to produce severe acne, arthrocele (joint swelling), disturbances in sight and hearing, jaundice, edema of the eyelids, and—most notably—a brown discoloration of the fingertips, nails, lips, and gums. Since 1969 in the United States, several instances of PCB-contaminated food such as milk, poultry, and cereal have been reported and have been attributed to accidental entry of PCBs into animal feed or to migration of PCBs from food packaging materials. In 1972 the Environmental Protection Agency ordered that PCB levels in waterways should not exceed 0.01 parts per billion and prohibited the use of PCBs as a component of food packaging materials.

316. The answer is D (4). *(Raffle, pp 663–669. Rosenstock, p 35.)* Fortunately, pneumoconiosis is usually a mild disease, which characteristically develops after 20 or more years of exposure to coal dust. It cannot be differentiated either clinically or radiographically from silicosis; both disorders are often present in the same patient. Development of progressive massive fibrosis (PMF), a disabling and often fatal complication, is uncommon.

317. The answer is A (1, 2, 3). *(Raffle, pp 706–708. Rosenstock, pp 26–27.)* Farmer's lung is caused by an immunologic reaction to airborne antigens from thermophilic actinomycetes found in moldy hay or grains (the same antigens also are responsible for the public health menace of mushroom compost worker's lung). To prevent molding, hay must be stored with a moisture content of less than 20 percent. Patients present with what looks like an acute viral infection, with fever, respiratory symptoms, leukocytosis, and pulmonary infiltrates. Later on, they may develop end-stage pulmonary fibrosis. There is no eosinophilia.

318. The answer is E (all). *(Benenson, ed 14. pp 46, 187, 214, 417.)* Farmers are likely to develop such disorders as histoplasmosis, leptospirosis, aspergillosis, and pulmonary disease caused by nontuberculous mycobacteria. *Histoplasma capsulatum,* a mycelial fungus that grows in soils around chicken houses, barns, and silos, can produce isolated cases of mycosis or an epidemic, the latter occurring when spores become airborne and widely distributed after soil is disturbed by farm machinery. While the usual reservoir of infection for leptospirosis is the rodent, some of the more than 120 serotypes of *Leptospira* can be transmitted to humans through contact with contaminated water, moist soil, vegetation, dogs, swine, and other farm animals. Some species of *Aspergillus,* including *A. clavatus, A. flavus,* and *A. fumigatus,* grow in farm soil, on plants, and in manure and can cause asthma, pneumonia, and otomycosis. *Mycobacterium fortuitum,* a nontuberculous mycobacterium that grows in soil, can produce a pulmonary disease similar to tuberculosis in humans and in other animals.

319. The answer is B (1, 3). *(Last, ed 12. pp 603–606.)* Differences in the biologic properties of inorganic and organic compounds of mercury have been learned through studies in Japan, Sweden, Iraq, and Pakistan—countries where many people accidentally have been poisoned by aryl, alkyl, and alkoxyalkyl mercury compounds. In contrast to inorganic forms of mercury, which accumulate in and damage the liver and kidneys, methyl mercury collects in nervous system tissue and causes mild to severe neurologic disorders due to atrophy of cells of the cerebellum and cerebral cortex. Nearly 90 percent of ingested methyl mercury is eliminated by action of the gastrointestinal system. The mutagenicity of methyl mercury has been demonstrated both in laboratory experiments using fruit flies and in evaluation of biopsies of persons exposed to very low levels of this compound.

320. The answer is D (4). *(Raffle, pp 499–511. Rosenstock, p 166.)* Skin exposed to freezing temperatures will first develop frostnip (freezing of the skin only). Skin with frostnip appears white and is anesthetic. If ignored, it will progress to true frostbite, which is characterized by freezing of the deeper tissues as well. The victim of frostbite should be moved into a warm room, and the affected part should be rewarmed rapidly in warm (40°C [104°F]) water. Pain during rewarming is common, but is not an indication for stopping.

321. The answer is C (2, 4). *(Braunwald, ed 11. pp 1069–1070.)* A common finding in people who have been exposed chronically to asbestos is calcification of the pleura and diaphragm. The pleural calcification is often unilateral. The pattern of calcification is unique and easily differentiated from that caused by trauma and surgery. Calcification of the diaphragm is so rare that this finding is almost pathognomonic for asbestosis. Bilateral fibrosis is not a specific finding to establish a diagnosis of asbestosis. Although pleural effusion is not specific, its presence in a patient with asbestosis should prompt a search for bronchogenic carcinoma or mesothelioma.

322. The answer is B (1, 3). *(Raffle, pp 513–515. Rosenstock, pp 177–178.)* Acclimatization to the effects of heat is usual. Heat cramps are characterized by short-lived skeletal muscle cramps, typically in the calf and stomach muscles. Heat exhaustion involves mental confusion, mild elevation of body temperature, and occasionally vomiting. In heat stroke, the heat stress has overcome the body's ability to control its temperature, which rises above 41.2°C (106.2°F). It is a medical emergency, and requires rapid cooling, intravenous fluids, and management of accompanying electrolyte abnormalities.

323.   The answer is B (1, 3). *(Last, ed 12. pp 899–901, 942.)* Deaths occurring in workers not covered by the Occupational Safety and Health Act (e.g., miners) and certain types of injuries (e.g., to cashiers during robberies) account for half of work-related deaths and injuries. Despite technical decisions and bureaucratic problems, this new regulatory framework has generated interest among labor unions and employers. However, a 1982 decision by OSHA administrators restricted the employee's right to know to the hazard, not the composition, of chemicals (this was to protect trade secrets). Although the process of regulating new hazards is cumbersome, by law the secretary of labor can enforce temporary standards for up to 6 months.

324.   The answer is A (1, 2, 3). *(Raffle, pp 240–250. Rosenstock, pp 206–207.)* It is important to distinguish between exposures to organic and inorganic lead because they cause different syndromes. Acutely, overexposure to inorganic lead causes abdominal colic and hemolytic anemia; chronically, it causes an insidious illness characterized by fatigue, depression, and a motor neuropathy. Overexposure to organic lead causes a syndrome limited to the central nervous system, with insomnia, anorexia, irritability, and, eventually, an agitated encephalopathy. It is usually seen in workers who have been cleaning gasoline storage tanks. Gasoline station attendants are exposed to an *organic* lead compound, tetraethyl lead (TEL), used as an antiknock ingredient in gasolines, although they rarely develop symptoms of toxicity from organic lead.

325.   The answer is A (1, 2, 3). *(Last, ed 12. pp 1278–1279.)* Once a back injury has been sustained, the muscles and ligaments of the injured areas are weaker than before the injury. Mechanical lifting devices should be used so that unassisted lifting can be avoided. Accident prevention programs should include consideration of a worker's physical condition and age as well as the frequency with which strenuous work is part of the work schedule. Back injuries often occur when workers do not readjust their grasp on a heavy, bulky load after it has been lifted. Preemployment radiographs are not helpful.

326.   The answer is B (1, 3). *(Rosenstock, pp 42–43.)* Occupational exposure to several metals, including arsenic, nickel, and chromium, has been associated with lung cancer. Other occupationally encountered substances associated with lung cancer include asbestos, uranium, and coal tar pitch. There are no known cancers associated with occupational exposure to either iron or silver.

327. The answer is E (all). *(Last, ed 12. pp 750–757.)* A sudden loud noise can cause a punctured eardrum, which may result in a hearing loss of 20 or more decibels if the puncture is large enough. Continuous noise can cause about twice the amount of hearing loss as intermittent sound, since intermittent sound allows the hearing functions some opportunity to recover. The greatest loss of hearing occurs in the first hour of exposure and then levels off. The spectrum of the noise is also important: at the same intensity, low-frequency sounds are less damaging than high-frequency sounds.

328. The answer is C (2, 4). *(Rosenstock, pp 23–24.)* Occupational asthma probably accounts for no more than 15 percent of cases of asthma in adults. All agents causing asthma appear to require an underlying susceptibility in the host. Diagnosis is made by history and demonstration of a decline of > 10 percent in forced expiratory volume in 1 second (FEV_1) during the work shift, recovery following change in exposure, or specific inhalational challenge.

329. The answer is A (1, 2, 3). *(Last, ed 12. pp 721–724.)* Microwave radiation, a form of electromagnetic rather than ionizing energy that has been studied since the early 1930s, can cause a variety of reactions in living tissues. When absorbed, microwaves usually induce hyperthermia: at short wavelengths (frequencies over 10,000 MHz), microwaves increase the surface temperature of, but are not able to penetrate, the human skin. At long wavelengths (frequencies less than 150 MHz), microwaves can easily penetrate through the skin into body tissues. At whole-body doses of 2,450 MHz (the frequency at which most home-use microwave ovens operate), effects in human single cells include protein coagulation and increased permeability of cell membranes.

330. The answer is C (2, 4). *(Rosenstock, pp 151–157.)* Only one in five cases of occupational contact dermatitis is due to an allergic response; most are due to a direct irritation by the offending substance. Allergic contact dermatitis, however, is a lifelong problem and will almost always recur upon reexposure. Chloracne, a particularly severe form of acne, is associated with exposure to halogenated hydrocarbons. It is occasionally accompanied by hepatotoxicity or peripheral neuropathy.

331. The answer is C (2, 4). *(Braunwald, ed 11. p 844.)* Diarrhea and excessive salivation are symptoms of parasympathetic overstimulation; in this setting, they would likely be caused by exposure to insecticides containing acetylcholinesterase inhibitors (such as malathion or carbaril). Poisoning with an acetylcholinesterase inhibitor is a medical emergency requiring appropriate reversal with atropine (2 mg given intramuscularly). In addition, if the poisoning is due to an organophosphate insecticide, pralidoxime (1 g IV) should also be administered. Phosphate binders, such as aluminum hydroxide, are used in the treatment of hyperphosphatemia and have no role in treating poisoning with acetylcholinesterase inhibitors. Taking a careful travel history would be unlikely to shed much useful information on the cause of excessive salivation and would simply delay appropriate diagnosis and treatment.

332. The answer is B (1, 3). *(Rosenstock, pp 110–118.)* Exposure to anesthetic gases has been associated with an increased incidence of spontaneous abortions. Exposure to cytotoxic agents, such as those used in chemotherapy, should be avoided during pregnancy. Pregnant women should avoid using *hexachlorophene*-containing soaps, which have been associated with birth defects. All personnel in intensive care units should wear lead aprons when there is portable radiography taking place, but there is no special risk associated with breastfeeding.

333. The answer is B (1, 3). *(Braunwald, ed 11. p 843.)* The heart and the brain are the two human organs that are most rapidly and seriously damaged by carbon monoxide. The entry into the bloodstream of small amounts of carbon monoxide is regarded as a serious hazard to health because the affinity between carbon monoxide and hemoglobin is about 300 times greater than that between oxygen and hemoglobin. The effects of acute intoxication by inhalation of air containing 500 parts per million (ppm) carbon monoxide include headache, impairment of mental acuity and muscular control, nausea, vomiting, and fainting. Inspiration for 1 hour of air containing 1,000 ppm of carbon monoxide usually results in convulsions, coma, respiratory failure, and death.

334. The answer is A (1, 2, 3). *(Braunwald, ed 11. p 1070. Raffle, pp 645–653. Rosenstock, pp 33–34.)* Silicosis, usually due to inhalation of quartz dust, is a chronic, nonimmunologic lung disease characterized by the development of pulmonary nodules, which may eventually coalesce to cause progressive massive fibrosis. Eggshell calcifications in hilar lymph nodes may be seen in about 20 percent of patients. Usually, patients have been exposed to silica dusts for many years. However, an intense exposure can cause an acute and fulminant form of silicosis, which can be fatal. Occupations at risk include mining, sand-blasting (sand is largely composed of quartz), construction, and ceramics. Workers die of silicosis with a total body quartz burden of less than 1 gram.

335. The answer is C (2, 4). *(Last, ed 12. pp 503, 901.)* More than 15,000 chemicals are used by industries, but threshold limit values (TLVs) exist for about 500 of them. Existing TLVs have been established on the basis of average exposures; thus, during the performance of a certain task, workers may be exposed at times to unhealthy levels of a toxic chemical. Furthermore, TLVs were established without consideration of the interaction of industrial chemicals and of the cumulative effect of exposure to these chemicals. The regulatory agencies have limited personnel resources and thus are unable to determine the degree of industrial compliance with all regulations.

336. The answer is E (all). *(Raffle, pp 591–593. Rosenstock, pp 167–168.)* UV-A consists of light from 320 to 400 nm and is often termed "black light." It stimulates melanin production and causes suntanning. UV-B consists of light from 290 to 320 nm and is found in both natural (sunlight) and industrial (arc welding) sources. UV-B light is especially hazardous when it lands directly on the eye, as when it reflects from snow. UV-C radiation (200 to 290 nm) is used in germicidal lights, such as those found in certain operating rooms. Both UV-B and UV-C cause keratoconjunctivitis: exposed workers should wear visors and special glasses. Although sunlight contains all three types of UV light, the upper atmosphere absorbs most UV-C.

337. The answer is A (1, 2, 3). *(Ingbar, ed 5. pp 417–431.)* Radioiodine (^{131}I), a beta-ray and gamma-ray emitter with a half-life of about 8 days, is excreted in the saliva, urine, feces, and perspiration of radioiodine-treated patients. The expired air of radioiodine-treated patients is not radioactive. Therefore, nuclear medicine and all other hospital personnel should avoid contact with soiled laundry, dinnerware, or flatware that such patients have used. Safety procedures for the handling of radioactive materials include the prohibition of smoking, eating, or drinking in places where radioisotopes are used.

338–342. The answers are: 338-B, 339-A, 340-E, 341-D, 342-C. *(Braunwald, ed 11. pp 1068–1075. Last, ed 12. pp 562–569.)* Occupational exposure to beryllium dust is a hazard to workers in the manufacturing environments of aircraft assembly, metallurgical processes, and ceramics. Focal, noncaseating granulomas are the consequence of long exposure to beryllium dust. These are followed by a diffuse interstitial fibrosis that reduces lung volume, decreases gas transport, and causes dyspnea and nonproductive cough.

Bagassosis is due to inhalation of spores of microorganisms, especially *Thermoactinomyces*. It is mainly seen in workers in the sugar cane processing industry.

The acute symptoms of byssinosis occur in many workers after years of breathing air containing dusts of cotton, flax, or hemp and consist of chest tightness, cough, and wheezing. In persons who have chronic byssinosis, the pulmonary damage is irreversible. Airways are severely obstructed and lack normal elastic recoil.

Rheumatoid pneumoconiosis, or Caplan's syndrome, is seen in coal workers. Progressive massive fibrosis, consisting of a network of reticular fibers and coal dust deposits, is accompanied by seropositive rheumatoid arthritis. (Although first described with coal workers' pneumoconiosis, seropositive rheumatoid arthritis has now been described with other occupational lung disease.)

Siderosis is caused by chronic inhalation of iron oxide dust that is airborne in the work environments of welders. Pulmonary tissue responses are not significant, but serious impairment of pulmonary function may result from fibrosis, the extent of which is determined by the silica content of the inhaled iron dust.

The most common inorganic dust–related chronic pulmonary disease is asbestosis, which affects not only the worker but also the family (e.g., from the person shaking work clothes) and the neighborhood.

343–347. The answers are: 343-A, 344-E, 345-D, 346-B, 347-C. *(Braunwald, ed 11. pp 610–613, 620–623, 738–739, 742–743, 1325–1335.)* Although most occupational diseases are not infectious in origin, it is important to be aware of those that are. Butchers, meat packers, farmers, and livestock handlers are at risk of developing brucellosis, a febrile illness caused by several species of *Brucella*, a gram-negative coccobacillus. Occupational infection usually results from inoculation through abraded skin or mucous membranes; gloves and goggles can prevent this form of spread. Infection may also result from ingestion of raw milk or animal tissues. Treatment is with tetracycline.

Sporotrichosis is caused by the fungus *Sporothrix schenckii*, a common plant saprophyte. Infection is usually caused by inoculation of the organism into a wound, such as that caused by a rose thorn. It usually causes a lymphangitic disease, with a localized papule and distant nodules. Treatment is with oral potassium iodide.

Air-conditioning workers and others (such as hospital patients) exposed to air from cooling ducts containing water are susceptible to legionellosis, a severe pneumonia caused by *Legionella pneumophila*. *L. pneumophila* is a gram-negative rod that inhabits warm moist areas, such as air cooling systems. It is named after a famous epidemic that occurred in 1976 at an American Legion convention in Philadelphia, in which at least 220 people were infected with a (then) mysterious illness. Treatment is with erythromycin.

Dentists and other health workers exposed to blood and other body fluids are at risk for hepatitis B, a viral infection. The incubation period is approximately 1 to 4 months. There is no treatment.

Spelunkers are at risk for histoplasmosis, a fungal infection caused by *Histoplasma capsulatum*. *H. capsulatam* grows in soil, particularly that enriched by bird or bat excrement (the reason it is found in caves). Infection, which is more common in the central and southeastern U.S., is usually asymptomatic but may cause a chronic pulmonary disease that mimics tuberculosis. Treatment is with ketoconazole or amphotericin B.

348–352. The answers are: 348-C, 349-A, 350-A, 351-D, 352-B. *(Rosenstock, pp 230, 247, 253, 174.)* Some of the new media used by artists today are hazardous materials that include solvents and paints composed of vinyl acrylic acid, vinyl chloride, vinyl acetate, ethyl silicate, and pyroxylin. Contact with and inhalation of such substances may cause dermatitis and systemic toxic reactions, respectively. These materials are especially hazardous if they burn; extremely toxic gases, including hydrogen cyanide, may be released.

The principal health hazard associated with pottery manufacture is due to inhalation of silica dust generated during crushing and screening operations. Workers in glass manufacturing plants constitute another occupational group chronically exposed to silica dust. The use of wet sand in the manufacturing process reduces the hazard of developing silicosis, but the hazard is still present.

Workers in many different types of unventilated settings, such as sewers and oil tanks, are exposed to hydrogen sulfide. This gas, which smells like rotten eggs, can cause blockade of cellular respiration in high doses.

In the production of molds and castings in foundries, the occupational environment is characterized by conditions of excessive noise, vibration, and heat, as well as air contaminants.

353–357. The answers are: 353-C, 354-E, 355-D, 356-D, 357-B. *(Last, ed 12. pp 587–615, 617–702.)* Of the 70,000 chemicals currently in commercial production only 1,400 (2 percent) have been tested for their carcinogenicity. Of these, about 30 have been found by direct observations of exposed human populations to cause cancer. β-*Naphthylamine*, an aromatic amine used to produce dyes, rodenticides, and many other chemicals, has been identified as an agent that causes bladder cancer. *Benzene*, or benzol, is used in the production of coal tar derivatives, solvents, paints, and printing inks, and as a cleaning agent by auto mechanics. Based on epidemiologic evidence, benzene is regarded as a causative agent of leukemia and lymphoma. Vapors of *nickel*, a component of many alloys, and nickel sulfides, when inhaled over long periods of time, have been cited as a cause of cancer of the nasal cavities and the lungs. The carcinogenicity of nickel is based partly on studies of nickel refinery workers, in whom these cancers developed more than 20 years after exposure. Also, workers in the *chromate*-producing industries are at high risk of developing cancer of the nasal cavities and lungs. *Vinyl chloride*, a gas at room temperature, has been shown to cause cancer of the liver, brain, and lungs. Skin cancer is induced by occupational exposure to arsenic compounds, soot, tars, and oils.

358–361. The answers are: 358-D, 359-C, 360-B, 361-C. *(Last, ed 12. pp 587–615, 617–702.)* Black lung disease, or coal workers' pneumoconiosis, is chronic fibrosis of the lung caused by inhalation of coal dust. The disease can be prevented by reducing levels of coal dust in mines. The United States Coal Mine Health and Safety Act of 1969 and the "Black Lung Law" of 1972 provide compensation for victims of the disease and their dependents.

Methyl mercury concentrates in red blood cells and in nerve cells and can lead to severe and fatal neurologic disease. Symptoms include paresthesia, ataxia, visual disturbances, deafness, personality changes, and spasticity. The largest known incident of methyl mercury poisoning occurred in the regions near Minamata Bay in Japan. Almost 4,000 cases have been identified, all resulting from pollution of the bay by effluent from local chemical plants, and consequent contamination of the bay's fish.

Sulfur dioxide by itself may not cause chronic bronchitis and emphysema. However, exposure to sulfur dioxide, in combination with suspended particulates and active chemicals in smog, has been associated with increased symptoms of chronic bronchitis.

Occupational exposure to thallium is associated with a characteristic triad: gastroenteritis, polyneuropathy, and hair loss. The neuropathy may persist. Most cases are associated with the use or manufacture of thallium-containing rodenticides, although thallium is used in several industrial and mining processes.

362–364. The answers are: 362-C, 363-A, 364-B. *(Rom, p 807.)* Acid rain results primarily from sulfur oxides and nitrogen oxides produced through combustion of fossil fuels and has gradually increased over the past 20 years. Acid rain has damaged lakes and forests in North America and Europe.

Burning of fossil fuels also increases the carbon dioxide concentration in the atmosphere. Because carbon dioxide absorbs infrared wavelengths of light, the earth is less able to radiate infrared light, resulting in an increase in the atmospheric temperature—the so-called greenhouse effect.

Chlorofluorocarbons used as propellants for aerosol spray cans may interact with sunlight, which results in chemicals that destroy the concentration of ozone in the upper atmosphere. The ozone layer blocks much of the incident ultraviolet light in sunlight. If sufficient depletion of the ozone layer occurs, the increase in ultraviolet light reaching the earth's surface may pose significant health hazards.

Mental Health

DIRECTIONS: Each question below contains five suggested responses. Select the **one best** response to each question.

365. The most prevalent mental disorder in young children is

(A) autism
(B) mental retardation
(C) behavioral problems
(D) schizophrenia
(E) depression

366. Depression can be caused or exacerbated by drugs used in the treatment of hypertension. Which of the following statements about this type of depression is true?

(A) More than half of all patients being treated with alpha methyldopa report depression
(B) Drug-related depression is often permanent, even if the drug is discontinued
(C) Most patients with drug-induced depression have an underlying psychologic cause of depression as well
(D) The prevalence of depression is related to the degree of lowering of blood pressure
(E) None of the above

367. The mental illness most likely to occur in young adults (ages 15 to 24) is

(A) schizophrenia
(B) affective psychosis
(C) involutional melancholia
(D) agitated depression
(E) none of the above

368. What proportion of the United States population is estimated to have a mental or emotional problem that requires therapy?

(A) 1 percent
(B) 5 percent
(C) 10 percent
(D) 20 percent
(E) 40 percent

369. Which of the following statements about the relationship between religion and suicide in the U.S. is true?

(A) There is no relationship between religion and suicide
(B) Catholics are at a higher risk of suicide than Protestants
(C) Catholics are at a higher risk of suicide than Jews
(D) Religious people are at a higher risk of suicide than those who are not religious
(E) None of the above

370. Infants born to mothers who are heavy drinkers are at increased risk of which of the following problems?

(A) Mental retardation
(B) Chronic liver disease
(C) Excessive birthweight
(D) Chorioretinitis
(E) Deafness

371. The highest prevalence of alcoholism is found among residents of

(A) rural areas
(B) small towns
(C) small cities
(D) the centers of large cities
(E) suburban areas of large cities

372. All the following are associated with the intravenous use of heroin EXCEPT

(A) depression of sexual drive
(B) anorexia
(C) viral hepatitis
(D) constipation
(E) convulsions

373. Which statement best represents a correct and generally accepted finding obtained in current epidemiologic studies of autistic children?

(A) Autistic children are most often members of lower socioeconomic families
(B) Autistic children are most often members of higher socioeconomic families
(C) Parents of autistic children are often emotionally frigid and introverted
(D) Autism is more prevalent among boys than girls
(E) Autism does not have a genetic cause

374. Which of the following is the most common infectious cause of developmental abnormalities in the United States today?

(A) Pertussis
(B) Measles
(C) Rubella
(D) Cytomegalovirus
(E) Toxoplasmosis

375. Which of the following persons is most likely to commit suicide?

(A) A 16-year-old girl
(B) A 65-year-old widower
(C) A 40-year-old married father
(D) A 30-year-old unmarried woman
(E) A 30-year-old divorced man

376. Suicide is the second leading cause of death in which of the following groups?

(A) High school students
(B) College students
(C) Blue-collar workers
(D) White-collar workers
(E) Housewives

377. Which of the following statements best describes the incidence of suicide?

(A) The peak incidence of suicide occurs in persons who are in their early twenties and then the incidence declines
(B) The peak incidence of suicide occurs in middle-aged persons and then the incidence declines
(C) The incidence of suicide increases directly with age
(D) The incidence of suicide decreases directly with age
(E) The incidence of suicide is equal at all ages

378. Which of the following statements about suicide is true?

(A) People usually give warnings of their intention to commit suicide
(B) Most suicidal people have formed a firm decision to die
(C) Once persons wish to commit suicide, they are suicidal for an extended period of time
(D) After persons have survived the suicidal crisis, the suicide risk for them is over
(E) If suicidal behavior is identified in a person, the same behavior is likely to be found in members of that person's family

379. Studies of the epidemiology of alcoholism have shown

(A) that it is often associated with a family history of strict abstinence
(B) that there is only weak evidence for a genetic cause
(C) that the usual age of onset in men is about age 40, during the midlife crisis
(D) that there is a secondary peak in incidence after age 65
(E) none of the above

380. Which of the following statements about alcoholism is true?

(A) There are about 30 million alcoholics in the U.S.
(B) About 10 percent of the population consumes 95 percent of the alcohol
(C) The incidence of alcoholism is highest among college graduates
(D) The incidence of alcoholism is about the same in men and women
(E) None of the above

381. In most states, the legal limit for blood alcohol concentration allowed for operating a motor vehicle is

(A) 50 mg/dl
(B) 100 mg/dl
(C) 200 mg/dl
(D) 300 mg/dl
(E) 400 mg/dl

382. Epidemiologic investigations of dementia have found

(A) that more than 90 percent of patients in nursing homes are demented
(B) that it is the most common cause of death among nursing home residents
(C) that more than 10 million persons in the U.S. have Alzheimer's disease
(D) that there is an increased incidence of Alzheimer's disease among relatives of patients with that disease
(E) none of the above

383. Which of the following statements about the use of nicotine-containing chewing gum to help cigarette smokers quit smoking is true?

(A) It is most successful in persons who are not addicted to nicotine
(B) It is most successful in persons with low levels of addiction to nicotine
(C) It is most successful in persons with moderate levels of addiction to nicotine
(D) It is most successful in persons with high levels of addiction to nicotine
(E) Its success is unrelated to the degree of nicotine addiction

384. Epidemiologic studies of homosexuality have shown

(A) that the prevalence of homosexuality in the U.S. has increased in the past 20 years
(B) that homosexuality is five times as common among men as among women
(C) that the overall prevalence of homosexuality in the U.S. is about 1 percent
(D) that there is an increased incidence of homosexuality among relatives of male homosexuals
(E) none of the above

385. True statements about alcohol include all the following EXCEPT

(A) one shot (1.5 oz) of 86 proof whiskey contains about 20 g of ethanol
(B) 12 oz of beer contains about the same amount of alcohol as 5 oz of wine
(C) 12 oz of beer contains about the same amount of alcohol as one shot of whiskey
(D) the rate of absorption of alcohol increases with carbonation
(E) the rate of absorption of alcohol is the same on an empty stomach as on a full stomach

386. The most prevalent psychiatric disorder among opiate addicts undergoing treatment is

(A) schizophrenia
(B) depression
(C) alcoholism
(D) antisocial personality
(E) mania

DIRECTIONS: Each question below contains four suggested responses of which **one or more** is correct. Select

A	if	**1, 2, and 3**	are correct
B	if	**1 and 3**	are correct
C	if	**2 and 4**	are correct
D	if	**4**	is correct
E	if	**1, 2, 3, and 4**	are correct

387. Correct statements about the statistics of suicide include which of the following?

(1) The mortality from suicide is highest in white males of all ages
(2) The incidence of suicide attempts is higher in males than in females
(3) The risk of suicide increases for several months following divorce, separation, or death of the spouse
(4) Suicide rates do not correlate with socioeconomic status

388. True statements about the relationship between mental retardation and ingestion of lead in the U.S. include

(1) there are about 2 million children at risk
(2) effects on the central nervous system are reversible with chelating agents
(3) diagnosis of lead toxicity is simple
(4) mental retardation is a late consequence of toxicity

389. Causative factors for organic brain syndrome that have been virtually eliminated as a result of the practice of preventive medicine include

(1) syphilis
(2) lead
(3) vitamin deficiency
(4) hallucinogenic drugs

390. The decline of the mental hospital as the focal or primary point for obtaining treatment was precipitated by

(1) the development of drug therapy that made the patient more manageable
(2) the belief that the longer patients were institutionalized, the less were their chances of recovery and discharge
(3) a change in a direction toward community-based treatment
(4) increased use of electroconvulsive therapy for depression

391. A patient presenting with new onset of mania should be questioned carefully about occupational exposures to certain chemicals, including

(1) manganese
(2) lithium
(3) carbon disulfide
(4) aluminum

392. The cost of alcoholism to society in the United States can be attributed to

(1) absenteeism from work
(2) increased accidents of all kinds
(3) increased crime
(4) increased morale problems of fellow workers

393. Important determinants of rates of death due to homicide in the United States include

(1) race
(2) age
(3) ethnic group
(4) sex

394. True statements about social determinants of health include which of the following?

(1) Divorced persons have greater mortality from cancer than do married persons
(2) Persons with few social ties (friends, activities) have greater mortality from coronary heart disease than do persons with many social ties
(3) Persons of lower socioeconomic status have greater mortality from diabetes than do persons of higher socioeconomic status
(4) After correcting for race and access to medical care, there is no relationship between socioeconomic status and mortality

395. Chronic barbiturate abuse is particularly common among which of the following groups?

(1) Elderly men
(2) Heroin addicts
(3) Unemployed teenagers
(4) Middle-aged women

396. Commonly abused depressants include which of the following?

(1) Methaqualone
(2) Phencyclidine
(3) Diazepam
(4) Methedrine

397. True statements concerning the use of depressants other than alcohol include which of the following?

(1) Barbiturates are the most commonly abused depressants
(2) Excessive use of depressants can cause physical dependence
(3) Barbiturates cause more accidental deaths than any other single drug
(4) Withdrawal symptoms usually are more severe than those resulting from narcotic withdrawal

398. The use of methadone in the treatment of heroin addicts is characterized by

(1) absence of an addiction to methadone
(2) half of participants leaving the program within 6 months
(3) high cost of the methadone
(4) long-lasting effects of a single dose (up to 36 hours)

399. Features that characterize families in which spouse abuse occurs include which of the following?

(1) Husbands of battered women have less education than those of nonbattered women
(2) Women who were abused as children are more likely to be abused by their spouses
(3) Women whose mothers suffered abuse are more likely to be abused by their own husbands
(4) Men who batter women are prosecuted in 25 percent of cases

SUMMARY OF DIRECTIONS

A	B	C	D	E
1,2,3	1,3	2,4	4	All are
only	only	only	only	correct

400. Differences in the reported incidence rates of mental disorders between various socioeconomic groups have been attributed to

(1) the more stressful conditions of life to which persons of lower status are subjected
(2) the bias of physicians who assign more severe diagnoses to patients of a lower than of a higher status
(3) the differences in perception of need for medical treatment of members of different social groups
(4) the variation in availability of treatment

401. The ratio of hospitalized to non-hospitalized psychotic patients is higher in lower- than in upper-class families because

(1) upper-class families are greatly reluctant to use state hospitals
(2) upper-class families have the economic ability to care for patients at home
(3) upper-class families make greater use of nursing homes
(4) the incidence of psychosis is greater in lower-class families

402. Characteristics of the type A personality include

(1) time urgency
(2) obsessive neatness
(3) excessive competitiveness
(4) inability to carry on a conversation

403. The incidence of anorexia nervosa has been increasing recently. True statements about this disease include

(1) it is two to three times more common in females than males
(2) there is an increased incidence in the middle and upper classes
(3) it usually involves a profound loss of appetite in its early stages
(4) its usual age of onset is in the teen-aged years

404. The mental disorders that appear to be more prevalent among males include

(1) alcoholism
(2) schizophrenia
(3) drug abuse
(4) affective disorders

405. The mental disorders that have their highest incidence in the geriatric population include

(1) involutional depression
(2) hysteria
(3) organic brain syndrome
(4) schizophrenia

406. Panic disorders are characterized by the sudden onset of overwhelming terror or anxiety. True statements about the incidence of panic disorders include which of the following?

(1) They are more common in women than men
(2) The usual age of onset is less than 15 years or greater than 40 years
(3) There is an increased incidence in family members of index patients
(4) They affect about 1 in 1,000 persons

407. Emotional disturbances of the postpartum period

(1) are more common after the birth of male children
(2) are more common with increasing parity
(3) rarely last more than 1 week
(4) occur in at least 20 percent of women

408. Parents who abuse their children are

(1) more likely to be alcoholics than are nonabusive parents
(2) found in all social classes
(3) more likely to have been abused as children than are nonabusive parents
(4) more likely to be men than women

409. True statements about the use of opioid drugs in the U.S. include that

(1) the highest rates of use occur among persons 15 to 30 years of age
(2) more men than women use opioid drugs other than heroin
(3) the number of male users of heroin is 2 to 5 times greater than the number of female users
(4) fewer than 1 percent of enlisted personnel in the military use opioid drugs

410. Stuttering is a disturbance of the normal speech rhythm and fluency and is characterized by

(1) an increased incidence in boys compared with girls
(2) an increased incidence among family members of stutterers
(3) an increased incidence in non-whites compared with whites
(4) an increased incidence among adolescents compared with younger children

411. Potentially preventable causes of organic brain syndrome include

(1) alcoholism
(2) pernicious anemia
(3) syphilis
(4) schizophrenia

412. Preventable causes of mental retardation include

(1) lead poisoning
(2) rubella
(3) phenylketonuria
(4) toxoplasmosis

SUMMARY OF DIRECTIONS

A	B	C	D	E
1,2,3 only	1,3 only	2,4 only	4 only	All are correct

413. Studies of attempted (unsuccessful) suicide have shown that

(1) it is 100 times more common than completed (successful) suicide
(2) about 10 percent of persons who attempt suicide eventually commit suicide
(3) it is most common in persons with obsessive-compulsive personalities
(4) it is more common among women than men

414. Population-based epidemiologic surveys in the U.S. using standardized diagnostic interviews have been conducted among adults ages 18 and over. According to the responses to these surveys,

(1) alcohol abuse or dependence is the most prevalent mental disorder among men over age 65
(2) about one person in five was affected by a significant mental disorder within the previous 6 months
(3) most persons affected by a mental disorder were receiving some sort of psychiatric care
(4) phobias are the most prevalent mental disorder in women of all ages

415. Studies of mental illness in college students have shown that

(1) the prevalence of schizophrenia is less than 1 per 1,000 students
(2) organic delusional states at examination time are usually caused by excessive use of caffeine
(3) suicide is the leading cause of death among college students
(4) adjustment reactions are the most common disorder that leads to psychiatric referral

416. The definition of alcoholism in the third edition of the *Diagnostic and Statistical Manual of Mental Disorders* (*DSM III*) includes

(1) the division of alcoholism into four subtypes: heavy alcohol abuse, probable alcohol abuse, alcohol dependency, and alcohol-induced impairment
(2) the use of the equivalent of a fifth of whiskey almost every day
(3) a duration of disease of at least 6 months
(4) an impairment in social or occupational functioning

417. Studies of the bipolar (manic-depressive) disorder have found that

(1) mania is more common than depression in men with bipolar disorders
(2) mania is more common than depression in women with bipolar disorders
(3) most persons present for the first time with mania
(4) the average episode of mania or depression lasts 12 to 24 hours

DIRECTIONS: The group of questions below consists of lettered headings followed by a set of numbered items. For each numbered item select the **one** lettered heading with which it is **most** closely associated. Each lettered heading may be used **once, more than once, or not at all.**

Questions 418–422

Dr. Vera Blues, a noted psychiatric epidemiologist, is interested in the diagnosis of depression. She develops a new test for its diagnosis, which she calls the Blues test. According to the gold standard, which involves meeting the DSM-III criteria, about 1 percent of adults in the U.S. are depressed. Dr. Blues studies her new test in 100 persons diagnosed as being depressed by the gold standard; 80 have a positive Blues test. She finds 400 persons who are not depressed; again, 80 have a positive test. She reports her findings in the Journal of the Society of Academic Psychiatrists (JSAP). Match the statements that Dr. Blues made in her article with the appropriate percentage.

(A) 80 percent
(B) 50 percent
(C) 20 percent
(D) <1 percent
(E) None of the above

418. "I found that the sensitivity of the Blues test was . . ."

419. "The specificity of the Blues test was . . ."

420. "The likelihood that someone with depression would have a positive Blues test was . . ."

421. "The likelihood that someone in the population with a positive Blues test would be depressed was . . ."

422. "The likelihood that someone in the population with a negative Blues test would be depressed was . . ."

Mental Health
Answers

365. The answer is C. *(Kaplan, ed 4. pp 1635–1690.)* Behavioral problems, including attention deficit disorders and learning disabilities, are the most prevalent mental disorders in children and occur in approximately 10 percent of children. Approximately 0.05 percent of children suffer from autism and 2 percent from mental retardation. Schizophrenia is a disorder that classically occurs later in life.

366. The answer is E. *(Croog, N Engl J Med 314:1657–1664, 1986. Wyngaarden, ed 18. p 289.)* Almost all drug-induced depression responds to discontinuing the drug. The prevalence is highest in patients using centrally active drugs, such as reserpine, methyldopa, and beta-blockers; up to 30 percent of such patients report symptoms compatible with depression. Although drug-induced depression can exacerbate underlying depression, it is most often seen in people who are psychologically healthy. There is no relationship between the prevalence of depression and the degree of lowering of blood pressure.

367. The answer is A. *(Kaplan, ed 4. pp 643–650.)* Schizophrenia has a high incidence among persons in their early twenties, while affective psychosis afflicts persons in their late twenties. The annual incidence rate for schizophrenia is approximately 1 per 1,000 persons in the 15 to 24 age group. Involutional melancholia and agitated depression are specific types of depression and have their highest incidence in middle-aged persons.

368. The answer is C. *(Kaplan, ed 4. p 309.)* The President's Commission on Mental Health estimated in 1978 that 20 to 30 million Americans needed some form of help for mental and emotional disorders. Studies of patients using medical facilities indicate that 1 out of every 10 had a mental or emotional disorder.

369. The answer is E. *(Last, ed 12. p 1391.)* The highest risk of suicide in the U.S. is found among persons who are not religious, or who practice Buddhism. Catholics and Jews, especially if they are practicing, are at the lowest risk. Protestants are at intermediate risk.

370. The answer is A. *(Kaplan, ed 4. pp 1022–1023.)* The fetal alcohol syndrome occurs in infants born to mothers who drink frequently and heavily during the pregnancy. Abnormalities in such infants include mental retardation, increase in perinatal mortality, microcephaly, short palpebral fissures, midfacial defects, abnormal hands and feet, ventricular septal defects, and hemangiomas. About 2 live births per 100,000 have the complete syndrome. Recent work suggests that occasional alcohol consumption during pregnancy does not substantially affect the fetus.

371. The answer is D. *(Kaplan, ed 4. p 1018.)* Most persons who have alcoholism live in the centers of large cities, and residents of cities of 50,000 or more are most likely to become alcoholics. Blacks in urban ghettos seem to be at particularly high risk. Medical students studying for Board exams are not generally considered to be at risk.

372. The answer is E. *(Kaplan, ed 4. pp 989–991.)* The use of heroin, while providing general stimulation, euphoria, and contentment, is associated with numerous side effects, including depression of sexual drive, anorexia, constipation, pruritus, insomnia, depression, death from overdose, and a variety of infections resulting from the use of contaminated needles (AIDS, bacterial endocarditis, bacteremia, infection with hepatitis B, and malaria).

373. The answer is D. *(Kaplan, ed 4. pp 1672–1674.)* Although in several early studies, the parents of autistic children were identified frequently as professional people or as having cold or obsessive natures, or both, these findings have not been substantiated in recent studies. In fact, autistic children come from all types of backgrounds, emotional settings, and socioeconomic levels; and autism now is thought to be caused by organic biological-neurological factors. Three to four times as many males suffer from the disorder as females.

374. The answer is D. *(Rudolph, ed 18. pp 566–567.)* Congenital cytomegalovirus (CMV) infection is the most common infectious cause of developmental delay and mental retardation. It affects an estimated 3,000 to 8,000 children in the United States annually. Immunizations against pertussis, measles, and rubella have almost eliminated these infections as causes of brain damage. Congenital toxoplasmosis is significantly less common than CMV infection, although it also can cause severe retardation and brain damage.

375. The answer is B. *(Kaplan, ed 4. pp 1312–1314.)* The incidence of suicide increases with age especially in whites. The highest suicide rate is found in the geriatric population. Married persons are less likely to commit suicide than single people.

376. The answer is B. *(Kaplan, ed 4. pp 1812–1814.)* Suicide among college students is thought to be second only to accidents as a cause of death. The risk of suicide is 50 percent greater for college students than for persons of college age who are nonstudents. One survey found that 35 percent of students at a state university reported symptoms of depression.

377. The answer is C. *(Kaplan, ed 4. pp 1312–1313.)* The incidence of suicide increases with increasing age; and the rate ranges from less than 1 per 100,000 persons in the age group 5 to 14 years to greater than 40 per 100,000 persons over 75 years of age. Suicide "attempts," however, occur mainly in young people, and the peak incidence occurs in persons who are in their late teens and early twenties. In the age group 6 to 17 years, 25 percent of self-poisonings are said to be suicide attempts.

378. The answer is A. *(Kaplan, ed 4. pp 1312–1313.)* Myths about suicide include (1) that people who talk about suicide do not commit suicide; (2) that suicidal people fully intend and have formed a firm decision to die; (3) that once suicidal, a person is forever suicidal; (4) that improvement after a suicidal crisis means the risk of suicide is ended; and (5) that suicide is inherited or exists in members of families. The facts are that (1) the majority—about 80 percent—of suicidal persons provide many clues and warnings about their intentions to commit suicide; (2) most suicidal persons have not decided to live or die and they assign their fate to the efforts or intervention by others to save them from death; (3) persons are suicidal only for a limited period of time; and (4) most suicides occur about 3 months after the suicidal persons have passed through their suicidal crisis. Finally, suicide is not inherited but is an act committed by individuals, is self-inflicted, and is motivated by many conscious and unconscious factors.

379. The answer is E. *(Kaplan, ed 4. p 1023.)* Alcoholism is four times more common in families with a history of problem drinking, even if the child was adopted out of the family. About half of all alcoholics have such a family history. There is also a marked increased risk in twins of alcoholics, especially monozygotic twins. The usual age of onset of alcoholism is between 20 and 30 years; it is rare for the age of onset to be after 65.

380. The answer is E. *(Kaplan, ed 4. p 1018.)* There are about 5 to 9 million alcoholics in the U.S. The incidence of alcoholism is higher among men than women; high school dropouts have the highest rate among educational subgroups. Persons with certain occupations, such as bartenders and musicians, are also at higher risk of being alcoholic. About half of the alcohol consumed in this country is drunk by 10 percent of the population.

381. The answer is B. *(Braunwald, ed 11. p 2106.)* Significant impairment of motor coordination can occur with blood alcohol levels of only 20 to 30 mg/dl. However, the legal limit in most states is 100 mg/dl (0.1 percent). Levels of more than 300 to 400 mg/dl can be lethal. Ethanol causes more cases of toxic overdoses than any other agent.

382. The answer is D. *(Last, ed 12. p 851.)* Dementia is an important public health problem, especially among the institutionalized elderly. Although about half of the patients in nursing homes are demented, coronary heart disease is still the most important cause of death in this group. The diagnosis of Alzheimer's disease, which afflicts about one-half million persons in the U.S., can only be made by excluding other causes of dementia. Alzheimer's disease is more common among relatives of patients with the disease, and among persons with Down's syndrome.

383. The answer is D. *(Last, ed 12. p 1023.)* Nicotine-containing chewing gum is a useful adjunct in helping smokers to quit. It is most successful in smokers who report high levels of addiction, but should be used in the context of a comprehensive program for cessation of smoking. Each stick of gum contains about 2 mg of nicotine, roughly the equivalent of one cigarette.

384. The answer is D. *(Kaplan, ed 4. pp 1056–1058.)* It is unknown whether the prevalence of homosexuality in the U.S. is increasing. Most observers believe that the prevalence is constant, but that increasing openness and acceptance have given the appearance of an increased prevalence. Surveys estimate that about 2 percent of women and 4 to 6 percent of men in the U.S. are homosexual.

385. The answer is E. *(Wyngaarden, ed 18. p 48.)* The concentration of ethanol is 5 percent in beer, about 12 percent in wine, and 43 percent in 86 proof whiskey. Thus 12 oz of beer, 5 oz of wine, and one shot (1.5 oz) of 86 proof (43 percent) whiskey all contain about 0.6 oz (18 g) of ethanol. A 70-kg man can metabolize approximately 9 g of ethanol per hour. The absorption of alcohol is increased with rapid gastric emptying, in the absence of foodstuffs, and in the presence of carbonation (as in champagne). Most absorption takes place in the small intestine.

386. The answer is B. *(Kaplan, ed 4. p 1001.)* About half of the men and 70 percent of the women undergoing treatment for opiate addiction suffer from a major depressive disorder. Other common psychiatric disorders include alcoholism and antisocial personalities. Schizophrenia and mania are rare (less than 1 percent).

387. The answer is B (1, 3). *(Kaplan, ed 4. pp 1312–1314.)* Completed suicide rates are higher in white males than in white females or in nonwhites of both sexes. The suicide rate increases markedly among elderly white males but not in females or in nonwhites. Males make fewer suicide attempts than females. Suicide rates correlate not only with age, sex, and race but also with marital status (the suicide rate is higher in single, separated, divorced, or widowed persons than in those who are still married), socioeconomic status (especially among poor, elderly white males), psychiatric history, and place of residence.

388. The answer is B (1, 3). *(Braunwald, ed 11. pp 852–853.)* Ingestion of paint chips containing lead, or soil and household dust contaminated with lead, is a substantial problem in children living in or around buildings that were erected (and painted) more than 30 or 40 years ago, when the use of lead-based paints was common. Diagnosis is easy: there are very high levels of free erythrocyte protoporphyrin (FEP), and the elevated blood level of lead confirms the diagnosis. The effects on the developing central nervous system are irreversible, but they may be the only manifestation of toxicity.

389. The answer is B (1, 3). *(Kaplan, ed 4. pp 851–870.)* In the United States today, organic brain syndrome from syphilis or vitamin deficiency is an unusual occurrence. (In the early 1900s, syphilis and vitamin deficiency were leading causes for admissions to mental hospitals.) However, many chemical agents, including lead and alcohol, are still causes of organic brain syndrome.

390. The answer is A (1, 2, 3). *(Last, ed 12. pp 1349–1354.)* A major impetus for the change from mental hospital to outpatient care was derived from the development of drugs that made psychotic patients more manageable and decreased the need for custodial care. The desirability of such a change was reinforced by studies in which investigators demonstrated that the longer patients were hospitalized, the more chronic their condition became. These demonstrations, together with effective drug therapy, led to earlier discharge from mental hospitals and outpatient treatment. Federal legislation supported the change by providing financial aid for community mental health centers. The use of electroconvulsive therapy has been declining.

391. The answer is B (1, 3). *(Rosenstock, p 142.)* Both manganese and carbon disulfide (an organic solvent) have been associated with toxic mania. That associated with manganese is known as *locura manganica* and is characterized by emotional lability and auditory hallucinations. Lithium, of course, is used in the treatment of the mania associated with bipolar disorders.

392. The answer is E (all). *(Kaplan, ed 4. pp 1020–1021.)* Major factors that contribute to the cost of alcoholism to society are absenteeism from work, decreased work productivity attributable to impaired abilities of the persons who have alcoholism and to the decreased morale of their coworkers, avoidance of work situations or activities that will uncover the problems of the persons who have alcoholism, increased accidents of all kinds, increased crime (about half of all convicted felons are alcoholics), and high personnel turnover. The problems of persons who have alcoholism extend to their families and friends and create the need for social and health care facilities.

393. The answer is E (all). *(Kaplan, ed 4. pp 1408–1411.)* Homicide rates are four times higher in the nonwhite population than in the white, twice as high in the age group 25 to 44 years as in the average of all other ages combined, three times as common in males as in females, and much more common in certain ethnic groups, such as Hispanics.

394. The answer is A (1, 2, 3). *(Last, ed 12. pp 953–970.)* Although there is an extensive literature on social determinants of disease, very little is known about how such factors work. Virtually all studies have found that four factors—female sex, being married, higher socioeconomic status, and a greater number of social ties— are associated with reduced mortality from nearly all diseases. These relationships are not altered by traditional risk factors (such as blood pressure), or by race or access to care.

395. The answer is C (2, 4). *(Kaplan, ed 4. p 1010.)* The groups of people who most commonly have problems of chronic barbiturate abuse are middle-aged, middle-class persons and heroin addicts who use barbiturates as a substitute for, or an enhancer of, heroin. Barbiturate abuse has been increasing recently among housewives. The most common pattern of barbiturate abuse among teenagers is episodic use.

396. The answer is B (1, 3). *(Kaplan, ed 4. pp 1003–1015.)* The commonly abused depressant drugs include barbiturates, methaqualone (Quaalude), and diazepam (Valium). In small doses, these drugs relieve tension and induce sleep. High doses, however, produce toxic effects, physiologic dependence, and withdrawal reactions. Metamphetamine hydrochloride (Methedrine), or "speed," is a stimulant, while phencyclidine (PCP), or "angel-dust," is a hallucinogen. In some cities, PCP has become so popular that PCP-related deaths outnumber those associated with heroin and barbiturate abuse.

397. The answer is E (all). *(Kaplan, ed 4. pp 1009–1011.)* The most commonly used depressants, especially among young persons, are barbiturates, drugs that depress the activity of several organ systems, especially the central nervous system, and can produce effects ranging from mild sedation to coma. The subjective reactions of pleasure and release from tension experienced by the user typically lead to psychological dependence, and all patterns of use are associated with real dangers. Both psychological and physical dependence result from chronic use of depressants and withdrawal reactions, lasting 3 to 5 days, are generally more severe than those resulting from chronic use of narcotics.

398. The answer is C (2, 4). *(Kaplan, ed 4. pp 997–998.)* The claim that methadone programs are the cure for heroin addiction has not been universally accepted. Continued use of methadone (Methadon) results in addiction; and, if not administered properly, methadone use can result in overdose reactions. Redeeming factors include a long-lasting effect and a low cost—about 25 cents per dose. A major problem with methadone programs is the low retention rate—only about half of participants remain in a program after 6 months.

399. The answer is B (1, 3). *(Kaplan, ed 4. pp 1092–1093.)* Only 2 percent of men who abuse their spouses are prosecuted. Although husbands who batter their wives are less educated than those who do not, educational status of women does not correlate with domestic assaults. Abuse of women in childhood is not associated with a greater probability of being assaulted by a spouse; however, women whose mothers suffered physical abuse are more likely to experience such assault.

400. The answer is E (all). *(Kaplan, ed 4. pp 265–273.)* The emphasis of early studies on the effect upon mental health of disorganized and stressful living environments contrasts with that of later studies in which investigators focused on factors outside the patient's immediate environment, such as physician bias, availability of proper treatment, and the effects of treatment on patients of different status levels. In their studies, Faris and Dunham in 1939 expressed understanding of the role that patients' knowledge of mental disorders and different tolerance levels played in bringing their disorders to the attention of medical professionals.

401. The answer is A (1, 2, 3). *(Kaplan, ed 4. p 268.)* Members of upper-class families attempt to keep their relatives who have psychoses out of mental, especially public hospitals, for upper-class families usually have the economic means and strong motivations to obtain home nursing care or the services of nursing homes for their relatives. Although the incidence of mental illness is inversely related to the level of social class, the higher incidence in lower classes is not generally considered by itself as the explanation of the higher *ratio* of hospitalized to nonhospitalized patients of the lower-class families.

402. The answer is B (1, 3). *(Kaplan, ed 4. p 1155.)* The type A personality was first associated with an increased incidence of coronary heart disease by Friedman and Rosenman, although that association is now controversial. They described two essential characteristics: time urgency and excessive competitiveness. Type B persons are more relaxed and less likely to exhibit goal-oriented behavior.

403. The answer is C (2, 4). *(Kaplan, ed 4. pp 1143–1144.)* Anorexia nervosa is characterized by altered perception of body image leading to severe weight loss. About 95 percent of the cases occur in females. Despite the name, anorexia (loss of appetite) is rare initially. Most cases begin between ages 13 and 16.

404. The answer is B (1, 3). *(Kaplan, ed 4. p 270.)* The prevalence of alcoholism and drug abuse has been shown to be five times greater among males than females.

While affective disorders afflict females at a rate about twice that for males, schizophrenia occurs in males and females at about the same rate.

405. The answer is B (1, 3). *(Kaplan, ed 4. pp 1953–1959.)* Involutional depression and organic brain syndrome appear during the later years of life. Hysteria most commonly occurs in adolescent and young adult women. The peak incidence for schizophrenia occurs in persons in the age group 15 to 24 years.

406. The answer is B (1, 3). *(Braunwald, ed 11. p 2089.)* Panic disorders are twice as common in women as in men. They are estimated to occur in between 1 to 2 percent of the population. Their usual age of onset is in the late teens or early twenties. There is a definite familial aggregation of the disorder, which is also sometimes seen in relatives of persons with affective disorders.

407. The answer is D (4). *(Kaplan, ed 4. p 1238.)* Studies of emotional disturbances in the postpartum period have found no relationship with sex of the child, parity, and a variety of other factors. Their cause is unknown, but is probably related to hormonal changes. Postpartum depression, the most common manifestation, may last up to 4 weeks. Between 20 and 40 percent of mothers report emotional or cognitive problems post partum.

408. The answer is A (1, 2, 3). *(Kaplan, ed 4. pp 1817–1821.)* Child abuse is a major problem in the U.S.—up to a million children are maltreated each year, resulting in from 2,000 to 4,000 deaths. Child abusers come from all social classes and educational backgrounds. The mother is more commonly the abuser, perhaps because of greater contact with the child. Abusing parents are usually psychologically immature and have poor impulse control.

409. The answer is A (1, 2, 3). *(Kaplan, ed 4. p 989.)* Three to four percent of young adults (ages 18 to 25) in the U.S. have had some experience with heroin. The male to female ratio, at least in urban settings, is about 3 to 1. Use of opioids other than heroin is also more common among males. Nearly 5 percent of enlisted personnel in the military reported some use of opioids in the previous 12 months.

410. The answer is A (1, 2, 3). *(Kaplan, ed 4. pp 1716–1717.)* The cause of stuttering is not known, but genetic factors are thought to be important. Stuttering is two to three times more common in males than females and is also more common among nonwhites. The incidence is highest in young children, although there is a secondary rise in middle-age. There is a strong family tendency to stutter: up to half of the relatives of stutterers have speech dysfluency.

411. The answer is A (1, 2, 3). *(Kaplan, ed 4. pp 873–882.)* Syphilis and pernicious anemia are clearly preventable causes of organic brain syndrome, syphilis through serological screening and antibiotic treatment, and pernicious anemia by recognition of the syndrome (B_{12} deficiency). Prevention and treatment of alcoholism have low success rates; however, thiamine supplementation may prevent Korsakoff's organic brain syndrome. Schizophrenia is a psychosis, not a form of organic brain syndrome, for which prevention is not currently feasible.

412. The answer is E (all). *(Kaplan, ed 4. pp 1646–1647.)* Lead poisoning and lead encephalopathy of children can be prevented by laws that eliminate or restrict the sale of lead-based paint, leaded gasoline, and lead in other products to which children are exposed. Phenylketonuria is preventable by mass screening of all newborn infants, followed by diet therapy if indicated. The congenital rubella syndrome is preventable by immunization of all children and of all susceptible women of childbearing age. Pregnant women should be cautioned about exposure to cat feces, which may contain oocysts of toxoplasmosis.

413. The answer is D (4). *(Kaplan, ed 4. pp 1311–1315.)* Attempted (unsuccessful) suicide is about 10 to 20 times more common than completed suicide. Only 1 to 2 percent of persons who attempt suicide, however, go on to commit suicide. Attempted suicide is most commonly seen in persons with hysterical or antisocial personalities.

414. The answer is C (2, 4). *(Last, ed 12. pp 1371–1373.)* A similar proportion (about one in five) of men and women surveyed were affected by a significant mental disorder within the previous 6 months, but the leading diagnoses differed by sex. Phobias were the leading problem in women of all ages, affecting about 10 percent. Problems with alcohol abuse were the most common problem in men ages 18 to 64 (affecting about 10 percent). However, over the age of 65, cognitive impairment was the leading problem (affecting almost 6 percent of men, whereas only 3 percent of men over 65 admitted problems with alcohol). The majority of persons whose responses indicated one or more mental health disorders were not receiving any mental health care.

415. The answer is D (4). *(Kaplan, ed 4. pp 1812–1815.)* Surveys have found that adjustment reactions are the most common reason that college students are referred to mental health services. More serious mental disorders, however, are not rare. About one in three students admits to symptoms of depression, and from 1 to 3 percent have schizophrenia. Suicide is the second leading cause of death, after accidents. Use of amphetamines commonly causes examination-related organic mental syndromes; excessive use of caffeine leads to nervousness and insomnia.

416. The answer is D (4). *(Kaplan, ed 4. p 1016.)* Alcoholism is divided into two subtypes in *DSM III*: alcohol abuse and alcohol dependence. Alcohol abuse requires (1) a pattern of pathologic use (such as daily use, or occasional excessive use);

(2) impairment in social or occupational functioning (such as an arrest for driving while intoxicated); and (3) a duration of at least 1 month. Alcohol dependence requires all the above plus evidence of tolerance or withdrawal.

417. The answer is B (1, 3). *(Braunwald, ed 11. p 2086.)* About two-thirds of persons with bipolar disorders first present with mania; of those, most have a predominantly manic course. Depressive episodes are more frequent in women than in men; manic episodes are more frequent in men. The average episode lasts 8 months. Patients average about 10 episodes in their lifetime, but the frequency of episodes increases with increasing duration of the disease.

418–422. The answers are: 418-A, 419-A, 420-A, 421-E, 422-D. *(Sackett, pp 59–100.)* Answering the first three of these questions is easiest if the results of Dr. Blues' research are displayed in a 2 × 2 table:

	Depressed	Not Depressed
Positive Blues test	80	320
Negative Blues test	20	80
Total	100	400

The sensitivity of a test is defined as the proportion of persons with a disease who have a positive test (positivity in disease = PID), in this case, 80 out of 100, or 80 percent. This is the same as the likelihood that a person with depression will have a positive Blues test. The specificity of a test is defined as the proportion of persons without a disease who have a negative test (negativity in health = NIH), in this case, 320 out of 400, or 80 percent.

The likelihood that someone with a positive test has the disease—known as the positive predictive value (PV +) of a test—depends upon how prevalent the disease is. By definition,

$$PV + \; = \text{true positives} \div \text{total positives}$$
$$= \text{true positives} \div (\text{true positives} + \text{false positives})$$
$$= (\text{sensitivity} \times \text{prevalence}) \div [(\text{sensitivity} \times \text{prevalence})$$
$$+ \; (1 - \text{specificity}) \times (1 - \text{prevalence})]$$
$$= (0.8 \times 0.01) \div [(0.8 \times 0.01) + (0.2 \times 0.99)] = 3.9\%.$$

The Blues test would not be very useful in diagnosing depression if applied to the general population. It might be useful in ruling out depression if negative, however. The likelihood that someone with a negative test has the disease equals 100 percent minus the likelihood that someone with a negative test does *not* have the disease. This latter quantity is known as the negative predictive value (PV−) and is defined as

$$
\begin{aligned}
\text{PV}- &= \text{true negatives} \div \text{total negatives} \\
&= \text{true negatives} \div (\text{true negatives} + \text{false negatives}) \\
&= [\text{specificity} \times (1 - \text{prevalence})] \div [\text{specificity} \times (1 - \text{prevalence}) \\
&\quad + (1 - \text{sensitivity} \times \text{prevalence})] \\
&= (0.8 \times 0.99) \div [(0.8 \times 0.99) + (0.2 \times 0.01)] = 99.7\%
\end{aligned}
$$

Since the likelihood that someone with a negative test is *not* depressed is 99.7 percent, the likelihood that someone with a negative test is depressed is (1 − 99.7 percent) or 0.3 percent. (A shortcut: Since we know that the overall prevalence of depression is only 1 percent, someone with a *negative* Blues test must be even less likely to be depressed than that!)

Community Medicine

DIRECTIONS: Each question below contains five suggested responses. Select the **one best** response to each question.

423. Compared with Western European countries (excluding Northern Ireland), the homicide rate in the U.S. is

(A) about 25 percent lower
(B) about the same
(C) about 50 percent higher
(D) two to three times as high
(E) about ten times as high

424. All the following statements regarding the trace element iodine are true EXCEPT

(A) adequate intake of iodine is essential because it is a component of several enzymes involved in intermediary metabolism
(B) deficiency develops primarily in areas where the level of iodine in the soil is insufficient
(C) it is extremely toxic at high doses
(D) deficiency leads to goiter, but rarely to hypothyroidism
(E) iodide supplements are recommended for persons who may be exposed to radioactive fallout

425. Which of the following statements regarding informed consent for medical treatment is correct?

(A) Physicians must disclose risks of a specific treatment, but are not required to discuss alternative treatments if they are less effective
(B) Because risks of procedures may be frightening, it is best to defer the discussion until after the patient has been sedated
(C) In order to be valid, informed consent must be written and include the patient's signature and the date
(D) The primary factor in the physician's responsibility to inform the patient of an adverse effect is the frequency of that effect
(E) None of the above

426. The parameter that can be used to obtain the best estimate of the prevalence of dental caries is

(A) the calculus index
(B) the malocclusion index
(C) the decayed, missing, or filled rate
(D) the oral hygiene index
(E) none of the above

427. Between 50 and 60 percent of fatal motor vehicle accidents in the United States are caused by drunk drivers, according to the Insurance Institute for Highway Safety. The most effective means to date of reducing drunk driving is

(A) heavy fine
(B) mandatory jail sentence
(C) rehabilitation program
(D) restitution
(E) suspension of license

428. What percentage of drivers killed in automobile accidents have blood alcohol levels above the legal limit?

(A) 10 percent
(B) 25 percent
(C) 50 percent
(D) 75 percent
(E) None of the above

429. Accidents cause over 100,000 deaths per year in the United States, and

(A) the death rates due to accidents are equal in men and women
(B) accidents are the most frequent cause of death in the age group 1 to 34 years
(C) half of accidental deaths occur in the home
(D) nearly 40 percent of accidental deaths occur at work
(E) fires cause most accidental deaths in the home

430. Carbohydrates are the least expensive and most easily digested form of fuel for human energy. Studies of nutrition and carbohydrates have shown that

(A) carbohydrates provide approximately half of the calories in the average American diet
(B) the consumption of carbohydrates per capita has increased in America since 1900
(C) fruits offer a more highly concentrated source of carbohydrates than do grains
(D) meats are approximately 20 percent carbohydrates
(E) milk is approximately 20 percent carbohydrates

431. In 1984, the highest infant mortality was reported for

(A) Finland
(B) Netherlands
(C) Singapore
(D) Japan
(E) United States

432. The routine clinical methods to detect obesity consist of the use of standard weight-height tables and the measurement of

(A) the specific gravity of the whole body
(B) total body water, using deuterium oxide
(C) lean body mass, using ^{40}K
(D) the thickness of subcutaneous folds of fat
(E) none of the above

433. The world population is currently estimated to be growing at a rate such that the number of years required for the population to double is

(A) 15 years
(B) 35 years
(C) 70 years
(D) 105 years
(E) 140 years

434. Mortality of whites and non-whites in the United States has been significantly different ever since data have been recorded. How much greater is the INFANT mortality for nonwhites compared with that for whites?

(A) 10 percent
(B) 25 percent
(C) 40 percent
(D) 65 percent
(E) 95 percent

435. In 1983, almost 1.3 million legal abortions were performed in the U.S. All the following statements concerning legal abortions are true EXCEPT

(A) the Centers for Disease Control (CDC) maintain epidemiologic sur-veillance of abortion in the U.S.
(B) the abortion ratio (abortions per 1,000 live births) has declined since 1980
(C) abortion related mortality was about 0.05 percent
(D) more than 90 percent of abortions were performed by curettage
(E) more than 75 percent of abortions were performed at less than 12 weeks' gestation

436. The total fertility rate in the U.S. in 1984 was approximately

(A) 1.2
(B) 1.8
(C) 2.4
(D) 3.0
(E) 3.6

DIRECTIONS: Each question below contains four suggested responses of which **one or more** is correct. Select

A	if	**1, 2, and 3**	are correct
B	if	**1 and 3**	are correct
C	if	**2 and 4**	are correct
D	if	**4**	is correct
E	if	**1, 2, 3, and 4**	are correct

437. Which of the following findings should raise the suspicion of child abuse?

(1) Multiple circular scars of approximately 1 cm
(2) Retinal hemorrhages
(3) Fractures of the femur in children not yet walking
(4) Multiple bruises of different ages over the shins

438. Overconsumption of refined sugar has been shown to cause

(1) obesity
(2) arteriosclerosis
(3) diabetes
(4) tooth decay

439. Correct statements about obesity include

(1) obesity is the major risk factor for non–insulin-dependent diabetes mellitus
(2) sedentariness is the most important cause of widespread obesity in Western populations
(3) obesity is a risk factor for coronary heart disease only among the extremely obese
(4) a woman whose body fat is equal to 24 percent of her total body weight should be considered obese

440. Correct statements concerning protein sources include which of the following?

(1) In the U.S. the majority of protein intake is from vegetable sources
(2) Proteins in eggs have the highest biologic value
(3) Wheat proteins contain adequate amounts of all essential amino acids
(4) Mixtures of vegetable proteins can provide all essential amino acids

441. Among the top five causes of death for adolescents (aged 15 to 19 years) in the U.S. are

(1) influenza and pneumonia
(2) suicide
(3) meningitis
(4) homicide

442. Diseases or conditions ranked among the ten most common causes of neonatal death in the United States include

(1) respiratory distress syndrome
(2) infections
(3) congenital malformations
(4) premature births

443. Correct statements regarding domestic battering of women include which of the following?

(1) Most instances of spouse abuse occur as isolated incidents
(2) Among married women, about 4 to 10 percent are beaten by their husbands over the course of a year
(3) The majority of instances of woman battering are caused by alcohol abuse
(4) Presenting complaints among abused women seeking medical attention are often nonspecific

444. Characteristic signs or symptoms of kwashiorkor include

(1) edema
(2) diarrhea
(3) hypoalbuminemia
(4) loss of subcutaneous fat

445. Correct statements concerning nutrition in infancy include which of the following?

(1) Protein requirements are greater in infancy than at any other time
(2) Human milk contains sufficient thiamine, niacin, and ascorbic acid to meet the needs of infants
(3) Iron deficiency is more common in infants and children under 5 years old than at any other age
(4) Human milk contains twice as much protein as cow's milk

446. Factors associated with maternal mortality include

(1) maternal age
(2) maternal race
(3) economic status
(4) abortion laws

447. Correct statements concerning iron requirements include which of the following?

(1) Iron requirements of women decrease after menopause
(2) Iron requirements are the same in adult men and postmenopausal women
(3) Iron requirements increase during pregnancy
(4) Iron requirements are satisfied by cow's milk

448. Major dietary sources of calcium include

(1) eggs
(2) milk
(3) beef
(4) cheese

449. Correct statements concerning breast-feeding include which of the following?

(1) The incidence of infections is greater in breast-fed than in bottle-fed infants
(2) Breast milk is frequently insufficient in quantity
(3) Iron deficiency anemia is less frequent in infants fed cow's milk than in breast-fed infants
(4) Significant quantities of immunoglobulins are provided by breast milk

SUMMARY OF DIRECTIONS

A	B	C	D	E
1,2,3	1,3	2,4	4	All are
only	only	only	only	correct

450. Correct statements concerning maternal and child health (MCH) programs include which of the following?

(1) The Women, Infants, and Children (WIC) program provides low-cost preventive health care services to women and their children
(2) Crippled children's services must be provided by the states, under Title V of the Social Security Act
(3) Funds for MCH programs remained stable under the Reagan administration
(4) Contraceptive services are among the most cost-effective public health programs

451. Correct statements concerning fluoridation of drinking water include which of the following?

(1) Fluoridation of drinking water reduces caries by about 50 percent
(2) The advisability of fluoridation is still controversial among dental public health experts
(3) The optimum concentration of fluoride in public drinking water depends on the average daily air temperature of the community served
(4) Fluorosis, a white or brown discoloration of the teeth from too much fluoride, is rarely seen unless the concentration of fluoride exceeds 6 parts per million (ppm)

452. Correct statements about obesity include that

(1) osteoarthritis is more common among obese persons
(2) in a normal person, 300 calories of excess carbohydrate will lead to the same weight gain as 300 calories of excess fat
(3) obese persons are significantly less active than nonobese persons
(4) the apparent association between obesity and hypertension is probably due to the use of inappropriately small blood pressure cuffs in the obese subjects

453. Since 1969, there has been a dramatic increase in the number of legally performed abortions in the United States. Characteristics of the majority of women who obtain abortions include that they

(1) are white
(2) are under 25 years of age
(3) are unmarried
(4) have had no previous live births

454. The number of acute illnesses and injuries requiring medical attention or restriction of regular activities in the United States in 1981 was 478 million, or 2.1 per capita per year. Which of the following accounted for more than 10 percent of acute conditions requiring medical attention?

(1) Dental conditions
(2) Common cold
(3) Headaches
(4) Injuries

455. Correct statements regarding casualties from nuclear war include which of the following?

(1) In the immediate postattack period, casualties due to blast and thermal injuries would predominate

(2) Long-term atmospheric effects ("nuclear winter") would be more severe if the attack occurred in July than in January

(3) A limited (100 megaton) attack on 100 U.S. cities would result in about 15,000,000 to 50,000,000 immediate deaths

(4) A major (6500 megaton) nuclear attack on the U.S. would result in few if any (less than 1 million) immediate survivors

456. True statements about marriage include that

(1) the ratio of marriages to divorces is 2:1

(2) the median age of brides is increasing

(3) an increasing proportion of 25 to 29 year olds are unmarried

(4) divorce is much less common among couples with children

DIRECTIONS: Each group of questions below consists of lettered headings followed by a set of numbered items. For each numbered item select the **one** lettered heading with which it is **most** closely associated. Each lettered heading may be used **once, more than once, or not at all.**

Questions 457–460

Match each set of symptoms and signs with the dietary deficiency.

(A) Vitamin A deficiency
(B) Thiamine deficiency
(C) Vitamin C deficiency
(D) Vitamin D deficiency
(E) Niacin deficiency

457. Petechiae, sore gums, hematuria, and bone or joint pain

458. Dermatitis, diarrhea, and delirium

459. Edema, neuropathy, and myocardial failure

460. Conjunctival xerosis, hyperkeratosis, and keratomalacia

Questions 461–464

Match each description to the proper trace element.

(A) Chromium
(B) Cobalt
(C) Copper
(D) Selenium
(E) Zinc

461. Works closely with vitamin E as an antioxidant

462. Cofactor for many enzymes; essential for normal sense of taste

463. Cofactor for vitamin B_{12}

464. Works with insulin allowing uptake of glucose; deficiency may lead to diabetes

Questions 465–468

Match each of the following.

(A) A private voluntary health agency
(B) A federal health agency
(C) A professional health organization
(D) An international health agency
(E) A health foundation

465. American Public Health Association

466. American Cancer Society

467. Pan American Health Organization

468. Centers for Disease Control

Questions 469–472

For each function or program select the responsible agency.

(A) Food and Drug Administration
(B) Federal Trade Commission
(C) Centers for Disease Control
(D) National Center for Health Statistics
(E) Environmental Protection Agency

469. Immunization and health education

470. Standards for drug manufacture

471. Guidelines of solid waste management

472. False advertising claims

Questions 473–476

Match the following.

(A) Hemolytic anemia in premature infants
(B) Hemorrhagic disease of the newborn
(C) Wound healing
(D) Rickets
(E) Polyneuritis

473. Vitamin C

474. Vitamin E

475. Vitamin D

476. Vitamin K

Questions 477–480

Match each disease or theory with the correct person.

(A) Ignaz Semmelweis
(B) John Snow
(C) Thomas Bayes
(D) Edward Jenner
(E) George Baker

477. Smallpox

478. Puerperal fever

479. Cholera

480. Probability theory

Community Medicine

Answers

423. The answer is E. *(Last, ed 12. p 1404.)* The homicide rate in the U.S. in 1980 was 10.5 per 100,000 per year, about 10 times higher than that in most Western European countries. For example, homicide rates in other countries were as follows: England and Wales 0.7, Netherlands 0.8, Iceland 0.9, France 1.0, Norway 1.1, Sweden 1.2, West Germany 1.2, Denmark 1.3, Northern Ireland, 4.2

424. The answer is A. *(Whitney, pp 451–452.)* The importance of dietary iodine rests only on its role as an essential component of thyroid hormone. The thyroid gland extracts the minute amounts of iodine in the diet for synthesis of thyroid hormone. If there is adequate iodine in the soil, plant foods (and animals that eat them) will have sufficient content of iodine. Seafood is also rich in iodine. If dietary iodine is insufficient, the thyroid gland enlarges (goiter) in order to be better able to extract the small amounts available. This generally allows the patient to remain euthyroid. The thyroid gland very avidly concentrates iodine, especially when the diet has been deficient. Because ^{131}I is a radioactive isotope present in atomic fallout, persons at risk of exposure to fallout (for example, Western Europeans after the accident at the Chernobyl nuclear reactor) may be advised to take iodide from existing (safe) supplies prior to exposure, so that if they are exposed to radioactive iodine, which has been shown to cause thyroid cancer, they will absorb less of it.

425. The answer is E. *(Hoekelman, pp 35–38.)* To make an informed decision regarding treatment, patients need to be informed not only of the risks of the treatment, but also of its expected efficacy, and the expected efficacy and risks of alternative treatments. Consent should be obtained before sedation, not only because the discussion should take place while the patient is lucid, but also because sedation itself may be associated with risks. Consent may be obtained verbally. As a general rule, the need to inform patients of adverse effects of treatment is more dependent on the severity of the adverse effect than on its frequency.

426. The answer is C. *(Last, ed 12. p 1475.)* The decayed, missing, or filled (DMF) rate is the average number of teeth per person that are identified as decayed, missing, or filled. The DMF rate is used to determine the prevalence of caries. The calculus index and the oral hygiene index measure the amount of plaque and debris formation. These indices are indirectly related to dental caries since plaque formation precedes the development of caries. The malocclusion index is a measure of the need for orthodontic care and is therefore unrelated to dental caries.

427. The answer is E. *(Trunkey, Sci Am 249:29, 1983.)* Efforts to reduce drunk driving through increased penalties, including mandatory jail terms, have been unsuccessful in the United States and Europe. Rehabilitation programs also have been unsuccessful. There is some evidence of a significant decrease in the rate of drunk driving arrests in a population when drunk driving convictions result in suspension of the driver's license.

428. The answer is C. *(Hanlon, ed 8. p 463.)* According to numerous studies, approximately 50 percent of drivers killed in motor vehicle accidents had blood alcohol levels over 0.1%. The automobile accident rate per mile driven for problem drinkers is twice that for nondrinking drivers. The probability for the occurrence of an automobile accident increases significantly with increasing blood levels of alcohol. For example, when the concentration of blood alcohol is increased by a factor of 3 from 0.05% to 0.15%, the probability that an automobile accident will occur increases by a factor of 10.

429. The answer is B. *(Hanlon, ed 8. pp 340–341.)* Accidents are the leading cause of death in persons aged 1 to 34 years and rank second in persons aged 35 to 54, fourth in persons aged 55 to 64, and sixth in persons over age 65. Accidents cause more deaths in males than in females except in persons over 85. Although nearly half of all injuries (most of which are not fatal) occur in the home, almost half of all fatal accidents are motor vehicle accidents. Occupational accidents account for slightly more than 10 percent of all accidental deaths. Falls account for 40 percent of accidental deaths in the home compared with 23 percent for fires.

430. The answer is A. *(Whitney, pp 38–39.)* Fifty percent of the average caloric intake of Americans is derived from starches and sugars. Although the total carbohydrate intake has decreased since 1900, the consumption of refined sugars has increased relative to cereals, grains, and potatoes. Fresh fruits contain 6 to 22 percent carbohydrates compared with over 60 percent in most grains; milk is 5 percent carbohydrates while meats provide negligible amounts of carbohydrates.

431. The answer is E. *(Wegman, Pediatrics 80:817–827, 1987.)* The overall infant mortality in 1985 in the U.S. was 10.6 per 1,000 live births: 9.3 for whites and 18.2 for blacks. This is much worse than Finland (6.3), Netherlands (7.9), Singapore (8.9), or Japan (5.5). In fact, the U.S. ranks 19th among countries ordered by increasing infant mortality. The high rate of births to teen-aged mothers may be partly responsible: the proportion of births to women under age 20 was 13.1 percent in the U.S., compared with less than 9 percent for all 14 countries with infant mortality less than 10 per 1,000.

432. The answer is D. *(Whitney, p 265.)* Use of standard weight-height tables and measurement of the thickness of subcutaneous folds of fat by means of calipers are routine clinical methods for detecting obesity. However, skinfold measurements correlate well with the more exact determinations of body composition obtained by whole-body specific gravity measurement, or by determinations using isotopic water or potassium.

433. The answer is B. *(Mausner, ed 2. p 250.)* The population of the world grew from an estimated two billion in 1930 to four billion in 1975. The United Nations projected in 1975 that the population will double again in 35 years, reaching a total of eight billion by 2010. However, the impact of birth control programs in China and other nations may alter this estimate.

434. The answer is E. *(Wegman, Pediatrics 80:817–827, 1987.)* The infant mortality for nonwhite (mainly black) infants is approximately 95 percent higher than that for white infants. The rates in 1985 were 18.2 per 1,000 live births in blacks, compared with 9.3 per 1,000 live births in whites. The reasons for this enormous discrepancy are not entirely clear, but lower socioeconomic status, later prenatal care, and more teen-aged mothers among nonwhites may explain much of the difference.

435. The answer is C. *(Centers for Disease Control, Abortion Surveillance 1982–83 [1986]: 7SS–9SS.)* Since 1969, the Division of Reproductive Health at the Centers for Disease Control (CDC) has maintained ongoing epidemiologic surveillance of abortions in the U.S. After peaking in 1980, at 359.2 abortions per 1,000 live births, the abortion ratio declined 3 years in a row to 348.7 in 1983. Seventy-six percent of abortions are performed in the first 10 weeks of gestation; 90 percent in the first 12 weeks. There are about 10 deaths a year from legal abortions in the U.S., for a rate of less than 1 per 100,000 (0.001 percent).

436. The answer is B. *(Wegman, Pediatrics 80:817–827, 1987.)* The total fertility rate (TFR) is an approximation of the number of children a woman is expected to have in her lifetime. It is calculated by dividing the number of births to women in each 5-year period between the ages of 15 and 44 years by the number of women in that age period, and taking the sum of these age-specific rates. In 1976, it dropped to a low of 1.768; by 1985 it had increased to 1.84 (1.75 in whites, and 2.20 in blacks). The TFR required for zero population growth is about 2.11.

437. The answer is A (1, 2, 3). *(Rudolph, ed 18. pp 760–764.)* Multiple, 1-cm circular scars may be the result of cigarette burns, an all too common form of child abuse. Retinal hemorrhages can occur from head trauma, and also from vigorous shaking back and forth (the ''shaken baby syndrome''). Any fracture in a child not yet walking is suspicious for abuse (with the exception of clavicular fractures in neonates and pathologic fractures due to bone disease). Bruises over the shins occur commonly from running and falling and should not in themselves raise suspicions of abuse.

438. The answer is D (4). *(Whitney, pp 624–626.)* Although sugar is popularly believed to be the cause of many ills, current evidence has demonstrated a causal role only for tooth decay. Like other carbohydrates, sugar is rapidly broken down to monosaccharides (glucose and fructose), so the metabolic effects are similar. Sugar is different mainly because of its sweet taste, and the fact that it is available in such pure form—unaccompanied by vitamins, minerals, or fiber. For this reason, excessive consumption of sugar may interfere with a balanced diet.

439. The answer is A (1, 2, 3). *(Last, ed 12. pp 1170–1171, 1231).* Obesity is the major risk factor for non–insulin-dependent diabetes, but it is relatively unimportant as a risk factor for coronary heart disease, except at extremes of the weight distribution. Obesity is commonly considered to be present when body fat exceeds 25 percent of body weight in men, and 30 percent of body weight in women.

440. The answer is C (2, 4). *(Whitney, p 104.)* Although in 1910 nearly half of the U.S. protein intake came from vegetable sources, now only about one-third is of vegetable origin. The biologic value of protein is the percentage of absorbed nitrogen retained by the body. It is highest for eggs (100), compared with fish (75 to 90), rice (86), or corn (40). Wheat protein is deficient in lysine and thus does not contain all the essential amino acids. Adequate mixtures of vegetable proteins can compensate for the various deficiencies in amino acids of individual vegetable proteins. The development of high-protein vegetable mixtures has been one approach to enrich the diets of people in underdeveloped nations.

441. The answer is C (2, 4). *(Hanlon, ed 8. p 421.)* The top five causes of death in adolescents are motor vehicle accidents, other accidents, homicide, suicide, and malignant neoplasms. However, the ordering of these causes varies markedly by race and sex. Nonwhites have much higher rates of homicide, while whites have higher rates for motor vehicle accidents. Overall, adolescent males have about 2.7 times the death rate of females.

442. The answer is E (all). *(Wegman, Pediatrics 80:817–827, 1987.)* Each year in the U.S. approximately 26,000 live-born infants die before they reach 1 month of age. In 1985 the neonatal mortality per 1,000 live births was 7.0. The leading causes of neonatal death include respiratory distress syndrome, infections, birth injuries, and congenital abnormalities.

443. The answer is C (2, 4). *(Last, ed 12. pp 1412–1418.)* In three surveys, the frequency of spouse abuse was 3.8 percent (in a national study), 8.5 percent (in

Texas), and 10 percent (a Harris poll in Kentucky). Spouse abuse most often occurs in an ongoing pattern. Although patients may present with specific injuries, often complaints are related to injuries incurred in the past and are not recognized by medical personnel as related to spouse abuse. Although alcohol abuse is associated with domestic violence, it seems to be more often the excuse than the cause.

444.   The answer is A (1, 2, 3). *(Last, ed 12. pp 1519–1520.)* Kwashiorkor results from a diet that is severely deficient in proteins and often sufficient or slightly deficient in calories. It occurs in toddlers after their weaning from breast milk to a diet high in carbohydrates and low in proteins and is characterized by changes in hair texture and color, ulcerated skin lesions, hepatomegaly, edema secondary to hypoalbuminemia, diarrhea, impaired liver function, and apathy.

445.   The answer is A (1, 2, 3). *(Rudolph, ed 18. pp 157–161.)* Daily protein requirements during infancy are 2.0 to 3.5 g per kg of body weight and are greater during infancy because the rate of growth is more rapid during this period than at any other time of life. Except possibly for fluoride, vitamin D, and iron, all the recommended allowances of nutrients are provided by human milk during the first 4 to 6 months of life of a normal, full-term infant. Iron deficiency is most common in early childhood, especially when cow's milk, a poor source of iron, is the major food source. The prevalence of iron deficiency anemia can be reduced by the use of iron-supplemented infant formulas and other infant foods. The protein content of cow's milk is three to four times higher than that of human milk; most of the difference is due to the larger amounts of casein in cow's milk.

446.   The answer is E (all). *(Hanlon, ed 8. pp 401–403.)* Maternal mortality is observed to increase with age, especially after age 35. These rates are nearly four times higher in nonwhites than in whites and also are higher among the poor compared with those of higher economic status. Availability of medically supervised legal abortions has resulted in a reduction of maternal death rates.

447.   The answer is A (1, 2, 3). *(Whitney, pp 439–450, 545.)* For adult men and nonmenstruating women, the recommended daily dietary intake of elemental iron is 10 mg. Menstruation increases the daily needs of women to 18 mg of iron. After menopause, the iron requirement for women becomes the same as that for men. Cow's milk contains little or no iron. Because the requirement for iron is high during periods of rapid growth (as in infancy), iron-fortified milk formulas or cereals are recommended for infants.

448.   The answer is C (2, 4). *(Whitney, pp 415–416.)* Milk and other dairy products are the major dietary sources of calcium and provide about 75 percent of calcium in the American diet. A cup of milk contains about 300 mg of calcium (almost half the recommended daily allowance), and an ounce of cheese about 200 mg, compared with about 27 mg in an egg and 17 mg in 3 ounces of chipped beef. The recommended daily intake of calcium is 700 to 800 mg per day.

449. The answer is D (4). *(Rudolph, ed 18. pp 158–159, 1019–1021.)* Colostrum and mature breast milk contain and provide to infants significant amounts of immunoglobulins, especially secretory IgA. The immunoglobulins, along with other resistance factors such as maternal macrophages, contribute to the lower incidence of infections in breast-fed compared with bottle-fed infants. Infants absorb more iron from human than from bovine milk. Cow's milk may also lead to iron deficiency by increasing occult gastrointestinal blood loss.

450. The answer is C (2, 4). *(Last, ed 12. pp 1709–1717. Williams, ed 3. pp 118–119.)* The Women, Infants, and Children (WIC) program provides *food vouchers* for pregnant and nursing women and children up to age 5. Eligibility is based on income (<85 percent of the poverty level in 1983). Funds for crippled children are administered through the states, with matching funds through the federal government, under Title V of the Social Security Act. Funding for maternal and child health was cut (by about 20 percent) by the Reagan administration, including funding for family planning, which is among the most cost-effective of public health programs.

451. The answer is B (1, 3). *(Last, ed 12. pp 1479–1486.)* Because of the consistent effectiveness of fluoride in reducing dental caries by about 50 percent, its use is now widely accepted among public health professionals. Controversy surrounding fluoridation is political, not scientific. The optimum concentration of fluoride in drinking water decreases with increasing mean air temperature because people drink more water when it is hotter. Moderate fluorosis occurs at a fluoride concentration of about 2 ppm; severe fluorosis at 3 ppm.

452. The answer is B (1, 3). *(Braunwald, ed 11. pp 1671–1673.)* Arthritis, particularly of the hip, is more common in obese subjects, probably because of mechanical stresses on the joints. Recent studies have shown that it is not only the number of calories consumed but their composition that determines weight gain. Normal subjects can compensate for excessive carbohydrate intake by increasing their metabolic rate. Obese subjects are less active than normal subjects, but the inactivity is probably at least partially a result, rather than a cause, of the obesity. The association between hypertension and obesity is real; it is not a result of inappropriate cuff size.

453. The answer is E (all). *(Centers for Disease Control, Morbidity and Mortality Weekly Report 35 (2SS): 7SS-9SS, 1986.)* The total number of legal abortions increased from 586,760 in 1972 to 1,268,987 in 1983. Death due to abortions (legal, illegal, and spontaneous) declined from 88 in 1972 to 11 in 1982. As in previous years, in 1983, 62 percent of women who obtained abortions were less than 25 years of age, 68 percent were white, 79 percent were unmarried, and 57 percent had never given birth to a live infant.

454. The answer is C (2, 4). *(National Center for Health Statistics, p 11.)* The leading causes of acute conditions in 1981, as determined by the National Health Interview Survey, were influenza (49.7 per 100 persons per year), the common cold (41.4), and injuries (33.2). These three accounted for 23.4, 19.5, and 15.6 percent of acute conditions, respectively. The incidence of dental conditions and headaches were 2.2 and 1.8 per 100 per year, respectively, or 1.1 and 0.8 percent of acute conditions.

455. The answer is A (1, 2, 3). *(Abrams, N Engl J Med 305:1226–1232, 1981. Daugherty, pp 207–232.)* Most deaths in the period immediately after a nuclear attack would be due to blast effects (e.g., the pressure from the blast knocking down buildings) and thermal effects (burns from intense heat generated by the explosion and from resultant fires). Estimates of immediate deaths range from around 20,000,000 from a "limited" (100 megaton) war to about 90,000,000 from a large (6500 megaton) exchange. Note that 1 megaton is equivalent to about 80 Hiroshima bombs. Immediate casualties, however, could easily be dwarfed by longer term problems with infection, famine, radiation, and ecologic effects. The ecologic effects depend on many factors, including the numbers and sizes of fires, deposition of their smoke, and season of the year. Nuclear winter effects would be much more severe in the summer because there would be less rain and snow to bring soot back to earth and because cooling of the earth's surface relative to normal temperatures would be much greater.

456. The answer is A (1, 2, 3). *(Wegman, Pediatrics 76:861, 1985.)* In 1981, 10.6 marriages occurred per 1,000 compared with 5.3 divorces. The median age of the bride had increased from 21.3 in 1963 to 24.4 years in 1982. The average number of children per divorce decree (0.94 in 1982) is similar to the average number of children in married-couple families, suggesting that couples with children do not have a lower divorce rate.

457–460. The answers are: 457-C, 458-E, 459-B, 460-A. *(Last, ed 12. pp 1520–1524.)* Scurvy due to *vitamin C deficiency* is characterized by pain and tenderness of the extremities, irritability, and hemorrhagic phenomena, all the result of defective formation of collagen. *Niacin deficiency* causes pellagra, which results in the four D's: disturbances of the gastrointestinal tract (diarrhea), of the skin (dermatitis), and of the nervous system (delirium and dementia). *Thiamine deficiency* leads to beriberi in which either myocardial disease (edema and cardiac failure) or neurologic signs predominate. *Vitamin A deficiency* leads to defects in epithelial cells of skin (hyperkeratosis) and to eye disorders (xerosis and keratomalacia, as well as night blindness). Vitamin D deficiency causes rickets in children and osteomalacia in adults; both conditions are due to the inadequate mineralization of bone.

461–464. The answers are: 461-D, 462-E, 463-B, 464-A. *(Whitney, pp 455–464.)* Chromium is found in food in several different complexes, including a small organic molecule called *glucose tolerance factor,* which seems to be important for normal carbohydrate metabolism. Deficiency of chromium impairs the action of insulin, and a diabetes-like condition ensues.

Cobalt's main function in the body is as a part of vitamin B_{12}, which is also called *cobalamine.* Deficiency syndromes linked to cobalt are those associated with deficiency of the vitamin. Chronic administration of cobalt can lead to goiter as a result of blocking iodine uptake by the thyroid.

Selenium is a component of glutathione peroxidase, an enzyme that works with vitamin E to protect cells from oxidative damage. The growth of human fibroblasts and other cells in tissue culture requires selenium. The metal cures or prevents Keshan disease, which is characterized by multifocal myocardial necrosis and endemic to Keshan Province in China.

Zinc is involved with many metabolic pathways, including those responsible for healing of wounds, sexual development, and taste. The developing fetus, pregnant woman, and growing child have higher requirements for zinc than do adult men and nonpregnant women.

Copper is important for formation of red cells and collagen, and for the function of the central nervous system.

465–468. The answers are: 465-C, 466-A, 467-D, 468-B. *(Green, ed 5. pp 409, 416, 420–422, 466–467.)* Professional health organizations are groups formed by persons who have met prescribed standards of training and certification and whose purposes are to promote the interests of the profession and to serve the public. An example is the American Public Health Association, founded in 1872, which establishes standards and guidelines related to public health, implements public health education through its journal, other publications, and meetings, and provides expert testimony to legislative groups.

The American Cancer Society, founded in 1913, is an example of a nonprofit, voluntary health agency, which was organized to disseminate knowledge about cancer and is supported by voluntary donations.

The Pan American Health Organization, established in 1901, is an international health agency representing the nations of the Americas. Its major concern has been control of communicable diseases. It has been integrated into the World Health Organization and serves as the regional office for the Americas.

The Centers for Disease Control, formerly known as the Communicable Disease Center, is a branch of the United States Public Health Service. It is the federal agency responsible for surveillance of communicable diseases in the United States.

469–472. The answers are: 469-C, 470-A, 471-E, 472-B. *(Green, ed 5. pp 71, 406, 409, 477.)* The Centers for Disease Control's responsibilities are to provide surveillance and investigation of epidemic diseases, to promote disease-control programs, to provide expert laboratory assistance to state and local health departments, and to promote immunization and health education programs.

The Food and Drug Administration (FDA) was established in 1906 to enforce the laws that regulated interstate transport and quality of drugs and food. The FDA, which received its current name in 1931, assures that safe and effective prescription drugs are sold to the public. To do this, the FDA tests products, sets standards for production and quality control, and judges claims of safety and efficacy.

The Environmental Protection Agency (EPA) is responsible for protection and promotion of environmental quality. The EPA sets guidelines for solid waste disposal, for hazardous waste control, for recovery of resources from wastes, and for the screening of potentially hazardous chemicals prior to production and distribution.

The Federal Trade Commission (FTC) is responsible for investigation and control of false advertising or labeling for substances hazardous to health, such as cigarettes and saccharin.

473–476. The answers are: 473-C, 474-A, 475-D, 476-B. *(Last, ed 12. pp 1520–1524. Rudolph, ed 18. p 1053.)* Vitamin C is necessary for normal collagen formation. Lack of vitamin C inhibits wound healing as well as causes scurvy. Numerous claims (each lacking substantiation) of benefits from vitamin E supplements have been made including prevention of abortion, prevention of coronary heart disease, and improvement of lactation. One of the few demonstrated vitamin E deficiency states is a hemolytic anemia that occurs in premature babies. Rickets results from inadequate vitamin D intake leading to failure of absorption of calcium and phosphate. Hemorrhagic disease of the newborn due to low levels of prothrombin and of other clotting factors can be prevented by administration of vitamin K_1 immediately after birth.

477–480. The answers are: 477-D, 478-A, 479-B, 480-C. *(Last, ed 2. pp 12, 70, 119, 122.)* Edward Jenner (1749–1823), an English physician, noted that dairymaids who had had cowpox never got smallpox and subsequently showed experimentally that inoculation with cowpox protected against smallpox infection.

Ignaz Semmelweis (1818–1865) was a Viennese physician who asserted that the cause of puerperal fever was failure of physicians to wash their hands on leaving the dissecting laboratory for the delivery room. Semmelweiss was ignored, but Oliver Wendell Holmes, the American physician, poet, and philosopher was effective in getting physicians to clean up their act when attending deliveries.

John Snow (1813–1858) was a London physician who found that cholera was much more common in houses served by the Southwark and Vauxhall Water Company, which obtained its water from the Thames downstream from London, than in houses served by the Lambeth Water Company, which obtained water upstream. He is famous for having prevented additional cholera cases by removing the handle of the Broad Street Pump, which was dispensing contaminated water.

Thomas Bayes (1702–1761) was an English clergyman and mathematician most noted for Bayes theorem, which describes mathematically how prior probabilities are affected by new information. Bayes theorem can be used, for example, to calculate the predictive value of a diagnostic test result, given the prior probability of the disease and the test's sensitivity and specificity.

George Baker (1722–1809) discovered that the cause of "Devonshire colic" was lead poisoning resulting from use of lead-lined vats to ferment apple cider.

Health Care Delivery Systems

DIRECTIONS: Each question below contains five suggested responses. Select the **one best** response to each question.

481. Which of the following statements about graduates of foreign (non-U.S.) medical schools is correct?

(A) Most foreign medical graduates in residency training in the U.S. are not U.S. citizens
(B) Foreign medical graduates account for about one-third of physicians in residency training in the U.S.
(C) About one-fifth of U.S. physicians are foreign medical graduates
(D) Less than half of foreign medical graduates are involved in direct patient care
(E) None of the above

482. What percentage of total expenditures for health care in the U.S. is paid by private health insurance?

(A) 10 percent
(B) 20 percent
(C) 30 percent
(D) 50 percent
(E) 75 percent

483. Health care expenditures in the United States have increased from $12.7 billion in 1950 to $387.4 billion in 1984. About what proportion of the gross national product was spent on health care in 1984?

(A) 2 percent
(B) 6 percent
(C) 10 percent
(D) 14 percent
(E) 18 percent

484. In 1984, $387.4 billion was spent on health in the United States. Approximately what proportion was devoted to (noncommercial) medical research?

(A) 2 percent
(B) 4 percent
(C) 6 percent
(D) 8 percent
(E) 10 percent

485. All the following are reasons for rapidly rising malpractice premiums EXCEPT

(A) investment losses by carriers of liability insurance
(B) payments of awards in installments rather than lump sums
(C) increased numbers of claims filed by plaintiffs
(D) increased size of malpractice awards
(E) the fact that new medical technologies raised expectations

486. All the following statements concerning diagnosis-related groups (DRGs) are correct EXCEPT

(A) they are the basis for prospective payment for Medicare patients
(B) patients are assigned to DRGs based on information from hospital discharge abstracts
(C) reimbursement for patient care provided is the same in different communities, and for teaching and nonteaching hospitals
(D) a problem with DRG-based reimbursement is that it provides a financial incentive to increase admissions of less ill patients
(E) DRGs have resulted in substantial reductions in Medicare expenditures

487. Which of the following statements regarding for-profit health care in the U.S. is correct?

(A) Psychiatric hospitals and nursing homes are much more often operated for profit than are general hospitals
(B) For-profit hospitals generally have lower costs than nonprofit hospitals
(C) After peaking in the late 1970s, the number of proprietary (for-profit) hospitals in the U.S. is decreasing
(D) Indicators of quality of hospital care, such as board certification of staff physicians and outcome of elective surgery, have generally shown that investor-owned chain hospitals are slightly superior to nonprofit or public hospitals
(E) None of the above

488. Which of the following categories of service accounted for the largest proportion of health care costs in the United States in 1984?

(A) Physicians
(B) Hospitals
(C) Drugs
(D) Nursing homes
(E) Dentists

489. All the following statements about physicians' incomes are true EXCEPT

(A) the median net income for physicians in 1985 was about $100,000
(B) the highest paid physicians are surgeons
(C) the lowest paid physicians are general practitioners and pediatricians
(D) after taking general inflation into account, physician income has not increased in the last 15 years
(E) physicians who have been in practice 30 years or more make less than physicians who have been in practice for 15 years

DIRECTIONS: Each question below contains four suggested responses of which **one or more** is correct. Select

A	if	**1, 2, and 3**	are correct
B	if	**1 and 3**	are correct
C	if	**2 and 4**	are correct
D	if	**4**	is correct
E	if	**1, 2, 3, and 4**	are correct

490. Correct statements about nursing home care in the U.S. include that

(1) mental or behavioral problems are present in the majority of nursing home residents

(2) about 20 percent of the population over age 85 are in nursing homes

(3) white women are the most frequent inpatients in nursing homes

(4) more than half of expenses for nursing home care is paid from public funds

491. Which of the following factors contributed to the increase in hospital costs over the past 10 years in the United States?

(1) Increased length of stay

(2) Increased cost of complying with regulations

(3) Increased numbers of hospital admissions

(4) Increased use of high-technology modes of diagnosis and treatment

492. Which of the following features led to the increase in the ratio of the number of physicians to population in the United States from 1965 to 1982?

(1) The Health Professional Education Assistance Acts

(2) AMA support of expansion of medical schools

(3) Immigration of foreign medical graduates

(4) The Hill-Burton Act

493. True statements concerning the physician population in the United States include which of the following?

(1) The majority of physicians today are specialists

(2) Young physicians are tending to settle and practice in the suburbs

(3) Physicians in highly populated areas do not tend to be primary-care practitioners

(4) The number of physicians per 100,000 population increased by 15 percent from 1965 to 1980

494. Statements that correctly characterize the operations of the Medicaid program include which of the following?

(1) Payments are made to providers of specified health care services for specified groups of low-income people

(2) Benefits are provided to recipients who meet eligibility criteria that have been determined principally at the federal level

(3) States must match federal funds to be eligible for the Medicaid program

(4) Program administration is primarily the responsibility of the Social Security Administration

495. Statements that correctly characterize the operations of the Medicare program include which of the following?

(1) Reimbursements are made to persons over 65 years of age for certain health care expenditures

(2) Reimbursements are made to persons younger than 65 years of age who are listed on state welfare roles for certain health care expenditures

(3) Reimbursement for hospitalization is based on diagnosis-related groups

(4) The program covers complete hospitalization costs for eligible persons

496. Payments for personal health expenditures can be grouped into two categories: (1) direct payments, made out-of-pocket by the individual; and (2) third-party payments, made by insurance companies, government-sponsored programs, or philanthropic agencies. True statements concerning sources of payment of personal health expenditures in the United States include which of the following?

(1) Government payments, as a percentage of the total, have more than doubled since 1940

(2) Direct payments constitute 50 percent of the total

(3) Health insurance payments, as a percentage of the total, have more than tripled since 1950

(4) Blue Cross covers over half of all persons insured for personal health expenditures

DIRECTIONS: The group of questions below consists of lettered headings followed by a set of numbered items. For each numbered item select the **one** lettered heading with which it is **most** closely associated. Each lettered heading may be used **once, more than once, or not at all.**

Questions 497–500

Match each description below to the proper health care organization.

(A) Professional Review Organization (PRO)

(B) Health Maintenance Organization (HMO)

(C) Independent Practice Association (IPA)

(D) Preferred Provider Organization (PPO)

(E) None of the above

497. Nonprofit association of physicians that reviews the quality of care provided to Medicare, Medicaid, and other patients

498. Group of providers that agree to provide services to specific groups of patients on a discounted fee-for-service basis

499. An organization that directly provides or arranges for all health services required by a defined population of prepaid clients

500. An organization that contracts with private physicians in the community to provide services to members of prepaid group health plans

Health Care
Delivery Systems
Answers

481. The answer is C. *(Igelhart, N Engl J Med 313:831–836, 1985.)* In 1983 the AMA estimated that about 21 percent of the nation's physicians were foreign medical graduates, and about 80 percent of these physicians were involved in patient care. In 1985 there were 13,451 foreign medical graduates in U.S. residency training; of these, 7,386 (55 percent) were American citizens. Overall, 18 percent of physicians in accredited residencies in 1985 were foreign medical graduates, but there was enormous variability from state to state: New Jersey (59.5 percent) and New York (37.9 percent) had the highest proportion of foreign medical graduates in their residency programs.

482. The answer is C. *(Levit, Health Care Financing Rev 7:1–35, 1985.)* In 1984, 31 percent of all U.S. health expenses were paid by benefits from private health insurance policies. Direct payments by patients covered 24 percent of expenditures for health care and philanthropic or charitable sources 3 percent. The remaining 42 percent came from public (government) programs.

483. The answer is C. *(Levit, Health Care Financing Rev 7:1–35, 1985.)* The percentage of the gross national product spent on health care increased from 4.6 percent in 1950 to 10.6 percent in 1984, after peaking at 10.7 percent in 1983. This amounts to approximately $1580 per person. About 50 percent of these expenditures were for institutional (hospital and nursing home) care, and 20 percent for the services of health professionals.

484. The answer is A. *(Levit, Health Care Financing Rev 7:1–35, 1985.)* Of the national health expenditures in 1984, 1.76 percent went to medical research, a total of $6.8 billion. The proportion expended on research had been only 0.9 percent in 1950. Following the establishment of the National Institutes of Health and the expansion of federal funding of research, the proportion of health care dollars going to research increased dramatically, reaching a peak of 3.6 percent in 1965.

485. The answer is B. *(LeMasurier, Health Care Financing Rev 7:111–116, 1985.)* Malpractice insurance premiums increased by 221 percent between 1975 and 1984, compared with a 107 percent increase in the consumer price index. There is considerable debate about the relative importance of investment losses and losses from paid claims, but numbers of claims and sizes of verdicts have been increasing. Payment of awards in installments, rather than in lump sums, has resulted in savings of up to 14 percent rather than increased costs to the insurance industry.

486. The answer is C. *(Igelhart, N Engl J Med 314:1460–1464, 1986. Stern, N Engl J Med 312:621–627, 1985.)* Diagnosis-related groups (DRGs) became the basis for Medicare reimbursement October 1, 1983, following passage of the Tax Equity and Fiscal Responsibility Act of 1982, which called for Medicare to develop a prospective payment system. Patients are assigned to DRGs based on hospital discharge abstracts, and the hospital receives a fixed level of compensation for certain DRGs. The compensation does vary somewhat from hospital to hospital, depending on wage costs in the community and whether the hospital is a teaching hospital, since teaching hospitals tend to care for sicker and more indigent patients. A potential problem with DRG-based reimbursement is that, because reimbursement is based only on the DRG, the hospital will make much more profit from hospitalizing patients with marginal indications for hospitalization. A possible benefit of DRGs is increased specialization of hospitals, so that hospitals will selectively provide the services they can provide most efficiently. Provision of services at low cost, however, depends not only on efficiency but also on case mix. Thus, distinguishing between specialization and "skimming" (selection of patients who will be least expensive to care for) may be difficult. DRGs have resulted in substantial cost savings: along with other cuts they have resulted in cost savings of about $40 billion between 1981 and 1986. While defense spending increased under the Reagan administration from 22 to 26 percent of the budget, Medicare declined from 7.6 to 7.1 percent.

487. The answer is A. *(Gray, N Engl J Med 314:1523–1528, 1986. Relman, N Engl J Med 303:963–970, 1980.)* For-profit health care in the U.S. has been increasing dramatically in the last 10 years, expanding from nursing homes and psychiatric hospitals, which traditionally have been more frequently proprietary, to general hospitals. Clinical laboratories, home care, and hemodialysis centers are also substantially for-profit industries. For-profit hospitals do not generally have lower costs than nonprofit hospitals, but collections per case from third party payers have been 15 to 20 percent higher in for-profit hospitals. Indicators of quality of care have not shown much difference between investor-owned hospital chains and nonprofit hospitals, although historical problems with proprietary nursing homes suggest that continued caution is indicated regarding quality of care in for-profit hospitals.

488. The answer is B. *(Levit, Health Care Financing Rev 7:1–35, 1985.)* Hospital costs accounted for 41 percent of national health expenditures in the United States in 1978, more than twice as much as costs of physician services (19 percent). The proportions of total health care costs devoted to nursing homes, drugs, and dentists were 8, 7, and 7 percent, respectively.

489. The answer is D. *(Owens, Med Economics, Sept. 8, 1986, p 168.)* According to a recent *Medical Economics* survey, the median income for physicians in 1985 was $102,520. There was a wide distribution by specialty, with neurosurgeons ($192,670), orthopedic surgeons ($168,750), and plastic surgeons ($155,000) at the top, and pediatricians ($79,110) and general practitioners ($71,540) at the bottom. Physicians' salaries have increased much more than the rate of inflation over the past 15 years, but older physicians have not kept up with younger physicians; median income for physicians in practice 31 or more years was only $79,950, compared with $121,890 for physicians in practice 11 to 20 years.

490. The answer is E (all). *(Last, ed 12. pp 1331–1335, 1650–1651.)* Mental and behavioral problems are the most common conditions among nursing home patients, with senility or chronic brain syndrome occurring in about 57 percent of patients. About 20 percent of the population over 85 live in nursing homes. The mean age of all nursing home patients is over 80 years, with only 10 percent less than age 65. White women are most likely to become patients in nursing homes because they have greater longevity than blacks and males. About 65 percent of nursing home expenses come from public funds, primarily Medicaid.

491. The answer is C (2, 4). *(Williams, ed 3. pp 189–191.)* Over the past 10 years there has been increasing use of x-rays, laboratory tests, and high-technology therapy. The increase in costs has occurred despite a leveling off of hospital admissions and shorter hospital stays. Some of the increase, ironically, is due to the cost of complying with regulations whose goal was containment of costs.

492. The answer is A (1, 2, 3). *(Williams, ed 3. pp 311–313.)* In 1965 there were 146 physicians per 100,000 population; in 1980 there were 199. The number of physicians in the United States increased dramatically after 1960 because of several factors. The AMA reversed its opposition to new and expanded medical schools, the Health Professional Education Assistance Acts of 1963, 1968, and 1971 provided financial support for new medical schools and expansion of existing schools, and immigration barriers against foreign medical graduates were relaxed. Increasingly, foreign medical graduates are U.S. citizens: 55 percent in 1985 as compared with 35 percent in 1979. The Hill-Burton Act provided federal funds for construction of hospitals and health care centers between 1946 and 1971 but did not stimulate an increased supply of physicians.

493. The answer is A (1, 2, 3). *(Williams, ed 3. pp 310–315.)* The physician maldistribution in the United States has been related to several factors including the decline in the number of general and family practitioners, a continuing trend for young doctors not to settle in urban areas, and the fact that the physicians who do practice in urban settings are not usually primary-care practitioners. However, there is not a physician shortage. In fact, there is increasing concern about a surplus: the

Graduate Medical Education National Advisory Committee projects a surplus of 70,000 physicians by 1990.

494. The answer is B (1, 3). *(Last, ed 12. p 1659.)* Medicaid provides federal funds on a matching basis to states that elect to enter the program. Criteria for eligibility to receive benefits and for the range of the medical services provided by the program are primarily determined at the state rather than federal level. Although legislative authority for Medicaid is derived from Title XIX of the Social Security Act, most program operations are carried out by state-employed administrators. States may impose copayments for optional services or for patients who are "medically needy" but have some resources.

495. The answer is B (1, 3). *(Last, ed 12. pp 1657–1658.)* Medicare provides reimbursement for certain health care expenditures for persons 65 years of age and over. Administration of the program is primarily the responsibility of the Social Security Administration. Providers of in-patient care are reimbursed based on which of 468 diagnosis-related groups (DRGs) best fits the patient's reason for hospitalization. Program coverage for hospitalization is not complete: the patient must pay a set amount per hospitalization (called the deductible).

496. The answer is B (1, 3). *(Levit, Health Care Financing Rev 7:1–35, 1985.)* Government payments (from federal, state, and local funding sources) composed 16.1 percent of total personal health expenditures in 1940 and 39.6 percent in 1984. According to recent tabulations by the Health Care Financing Administration, direct payments constituted 27.9 percent of the $1580 per capita cost of personal health care in 1984. Health insurance payments as a percentage of the total have more than tripled from about 9 percent in 1950 to about 31 percent in 1984. While Blue Cross is the largest single insurer for personal health expenses, commercial carriers and independent plans have almost twice as many total enrollees as Blue Cross (145 million to 79 million).

497–500. The answers are: 497-A, 498-D, 499-B, 500-C. *(Mayer, N Engl J Med 312:590–594, 1985. Williams, ed 3. pp 144–147, 365, 395.)* Review of the quality of care is the purview of Professional Review Organizations (PROs), formerly called Professional Standards Review Organizations, which were established in the 1972 Social Security Amendments. PROs may contract with businesses as well as with the Department of Health and Human Services (DHHS) to monitor quality of care and hospital utilization.

Preferred Provider Organizations (PPOs) are groups of providers that make special arrangements with insurers to provide services to their customers on a discounted basis, i.e., to accept lower levels of reimbursement than their usual rates. An example is the Blue Cross "Prudent Buyer Plan," in which patients who are willing to obtain care from preferred providers can save on coinsurance and de-ductibles.

Health Maintenance Organizations (HMOs) provide comprehensive health care services on a prepaid basis. First developed around the turn of the century, they were bitterly opposed by organized medicine. In the early 1970s, legislation en-couraging their development was passed, which led to the establishment of 166 HMOs by 1975 and to 323 HMOs covering 15 million members by 1985.

Independent Practice Associations (IPAs) are a more recent development. Whereas HMOs have traditionally served their patients by employing full-time phy-sicians in their own clinics and medical centers, IPAs allow private physicians to contract with HMOs to provide services to enrolled patients.

Bibliography

Abrams HL, Van Kaenel WE: Medical problems of survivors of nuclear war. *N Engl J Med* 305:1226–1232, 1981.

American Academy of Pediatrics: *Report of the Committee on Infectious Disease.* American Academy of Pediatrics, Evanston, Illinois, 1986.

Benenson AS (ed): *Control of Communicable Disease in Man,* 14th ed. Washington, American Public Health Association Publications, 1985.

Brandenburg, K, Deinard AS, DiNapoli J, et al: 1% permethrin cream rinse vs 1% lindane shampoo in treating pediculosis capitis. *Am J Dis Child* 140:894–896, 1986.

Braunwald E, Isselbacher KJ, Petersdorf RG, et al (eds): *Harrison's Principles of Internal Medicine,* 11th ed. New York, McGraw-Hill, 1987.

Browner WS, Newman TB: Are all significant p values created equal? The analogy between diagnostic tests and clinical research. *JAMA* 257:2459–2463, 1987.

California Department of Health Services, Infectious Disease Branch: The significance and accuracy of ELISA tests for HIV antibodies. *California Morbidity* no. 44, 1986.

Centers for Disease Control: *Immunization Against Disease.* Atlanta, U.S. Department of Health and Human Services, 1983.

Centers for Disease Control: *State Immunization Requirements for School Children.* Atlanta, U.S. Department of Health and Human Services, 1983.

Centers for Disease Control: Abortion surveillance: Preliminary analysis, United States, 1982–1983. *Morbidity and Mortality Weekly Report Surveillance Summaries* 35(2SS): 7SS–9SS, 1986.

Centers for Disease Control: Influenza activity in civilian and military populations, and key points for use of influenza vaccines. *Morbidity and Mortality Weekly Report* 35:729–731, 1986.

Centers for Disease Control: Influenza vaccines, 1983–1984. *Morbidity and Mortality Weekly Report* 32:333–337, 1983.

Cherry, JD, Brunell PA, Golden GS, Karzon DT: Report of the task force on pertussis and pertussis immunization—1988. *Pediatrics* 81:939–984, 1988.

Colton T: *Statistics in Medicine.* Boston, Little, Brown, 1974.

Croog S, Levine S, Testa M, et al: The effects of antihypertensive therapy on the quality of life. *N Engl J Med* 314: 1657–1664, 1986.

Daugherty W, Levi B, Von Hippel F: Casualties due to the blast, heat, and radioactive fallout from various hypothetical nuclear attacks on the United States. In *The Medical Implications of Nuclear War,* Solomon F and Marston RQ, eds. Washington, DC, National Academy Press, 1986, pp 207–232.

187

Ehrlich O, Brem AS: A prospective comparison of urinary tract infections in patients treated with either clean intermittent catheterization or urinary diversion. *Pediatrics* 70:665, 1982.

Expert Panel: Report of the National Cholesterol Education Program Expert Panel on the detection, evaluation and treatment of high blood cholesterol in adults. *Arch Intern Med* 148:37–69, 1988.

Fauci A, Macher AM, Longgo DL, et al: Acquired immunodeficiency syndrome: Epidemiologic, clinical, immunologic, and therapeutic considerations. *Ann Intern Med* 100:92–106, 1984.

Feigin, RD, and Cherry, JD: *Textbook of Pediatric Infectious Disease,* 2nd ed. Philadelphia, WB Saunders, 1987.

Francis DP, Petricciani JC: The prospects for and pathways towards a vaccine for AIDS. *N Engl J Med* 313: 1586–1590, 1985.

Friedland GH, Klein RS: Transmission of the human immunodeficiency virus. *N Engl J Med* 317:1125–1135, 1987.

Gray BH, McNerney MHA: For-profit enterprise in health care: The Institute of Medicine study. *N Engl J Med* 314:1523–1528, 1986.

Greaves WL, Orenstein WA, Hinman AR, et al: Clinical efficacy of rubella vaccine. *Pediatr Infect Dis* 2:284–286, 1983.

Green LW, Anderson CL: *Community Health.* 5th ed. St. Louis, CV Mosby, 1985.

Hanlon JJ, Pickett GE: *Public Health: Administration and Practice,* 8th ed. St. Louis, CV Mosby, 1984.

Hearst N, Hulley SB: Preventing the heterosexual spread of AIDS: Are we giving our patients the best advice? *JAMA* 259:2428–2432, 1988.

Hoekelman RA, Blatman S, Friedman SB, et al: *Primary Pediatric Care.* St. Louis, CV Mosby, 1987.

Hulley SB, Cummings S (eds): *Designing Clinical Research: An Epidemiologic Approach.* Baltimore, Williams & Wilkins, 1988.

Igelhart JK: Reducing residency opportunities for graduates of foreign medical schools. *N Engl J Med* 313:831–836, 1985.

Igelhart JK: Early experience with prospective payment of hospitals. *N Engl J Med* 314:1460–1464, 1986.

Ingbar SH, Braverman LE: *Werner's The Thyroid,* 5th ed. Philadelphia, JB Lippincott, 1986.

Ingelfinger JA, Mosteller F, Thibodeau LA, Ware JH: *Biostatistics in Clinical Medicine,* 2nd ed. New York, Macmillan, 1986.

Kaplan, HI, Sadock BJ: *Comprehensive Textbook of Psychiatry*, 4th ed. Baltimore, Williams & Wilkins, 1985.

Last JM (ed): *A Dictionary of Epidemiology*, 2nd ed. New York, Oxford University Press, 1988.

Last JM: *Maxcy-Rosenau Preventive Medicine and Public Health*, 12th ed. New York, Prentice-Hall, Appleton-Century-Crofts, 1986.

LeMasurier J: Physician medical malpractice. *Health Care Financing Rev* 7:111–116, 1985.

Levit KR, Lazenby H, Waldo DR, Davidoff LM: National health expenditures, 1984. *Health Care Financing Rev* 7:1–35, 1985.

Lilienfeld AM, Lilienfeld DE: *Foundations of Epidemiology*, 2nd ed. New York, Oxford University Press, 1980.

Mandell LA, Ralph ED: *Essentials of Infectious Diseases*. Boston, Blackwell Scientific Publications, 1985.

Mausner JS, Kramer S: *Mausner and Bahn Epidemiology: An Introductory Text*, 2nd ed. Philadelphia, WB Saunders, 1985.

Mayer TR, Mayer GG: HMOs: Origins and development. *N Engl J Med* 312:590–594, 1985.

Michael M, Boyce WT, Wilcox AJ: *Biomedical Bestiary: An Epidemiologic Guide to Flaws and Fallacies in the Medical Literature*. Boston, Little, Brown, 1985.

National Center for Health Statistics: *Physicians' Handbook on Medical Certification: Death, Birth, Fetal Death*. Publication No. (PHS) 78-1108. Hyattsville, United States Department of Health, Education and Welfare, 1978.

National Center for Health Statistics: Current estimates from the national health interview survey, United States, 1981. *Vital and Health Statistics*, ser. 10, no. 141. DHHS Pub. No. (PHS) 83–1569. Washington, DC, Public Health Service, U.S. Government Printing Office, 1982.

Owens A: Earnings: Have they flattened out? Med Economics, Sept. 8, 1986, p 168.

Page JD: *Psychopathology: The Science of Understanding Deviance*, 3rd ed. Chicago, Aldine Publishing, 1975.

Page HS, Asire AJ: Cancer Rates and Risks, 3rd ed. Washington, DC, U.S. Department of Health and Human Services, NIH Pub. no. 85–691, 1985.

Pickering LK. Engelkirk PG: Giardia lamblia. *Pediatr Clin North Am* 35:565–577, 1988.

Raffle PAB, Lee WR, McCallum RI, Murray R (eds): *Hunter's Diseases of Occupations*. Boston, Little, Brown, 1987.

Relman AS: The new medical-industrial complex. *N Engl J Med* 303:963–970, 1980.

Remington JS, Klein JO: *Infectious Diseases of the Fetus and Newborn Infant,* 2nd ed. Philadelphia, WB Saunders, 1983.

Robbins SL, Cotran RS, Kumar V: *Pathologic Basis of Disease,* 3rd ed. Philadelphia, WB Saunders, 1984.

Rom WN (ed): *Environmental and Occupational Medicine.* Boston, Little, Brown, 1983.

Rosenstock L, Cullen MR: *Clinical Occupational Medicine.* Philadelphia, WB Saunders, 1986.

Rothman KJ: *Modern Epidemiology.* Boston, Little, Brown, 1986.

Rudolph AM, et al (eds): *Pediatrics,* 18th ed. New York, Prentice-Hall, Appleton-Century-Crofts, 1987.

Sackett DL, Haynes RB, Tugwell P: *Clinical Epidemiology: A Basic Science for Clinical Medicine.* Boston, Little, Brown, 1985.

Schlesselman JJ, Stolley PD: *Case Control Studies: Design, Conduct, Analysis.* New York, Oxford University Press, 1982.

Schottenfeld D, Fraumeni JF Jr: *Cancer Epidemiology and Prevention.* Philadelphia, WB Saunders, 1982.

Siegel AF: *Statistics and Data Analysis: An Introduction.* New York, John Wiley & Sons, 1988.

Stern RS, Epstein AM: Institutional responses to prospective payment based on diagnosis-related groups. Implications for cost, quality, and access. *N Engl J Med* 312:621–627, 1985.

Trunkey DD: Trauma. *Scientific American* 249:28–35, 1983.

Wegman ME: Annual summary of vital statistics, 1984. *Pediatrics* 76:861, 1985.

Wegman ME: Annual summary of vital statistics, 1986. *Pediatrics* 80:817–827, 1987.

Whitney EN, Cataldo CB: *Understanding Normal and Clinical Nutrition.* St. Paul, MN, West Publishing, 1983.

Williams SJ, Torrens PR (eds): *Introduction to Health Services,* 3rd ed. New York, John Wiley & Sons, 1988.

Wyngaarden JB, Smith LH Jr: *Cecil Textbook of Medicine,* 18th ed. Philadelphia, WB Saunders, 1988.